Contributors

Patricia M. Feeney, RN, BSN, MSW
Freelance writer and Public Relations consultant
St. Louis, Missouri

Lynda Hilliard, MBA, RN, CNAA
Director of Ancillary Services
Delta Memorial Hospital (Sutter Health Affiliate)
Antioch, California

Elizabeth Hogue, JD
Attorney, private practice
Silver Spring, Maryland

T. M. Marrelli, RN, MA
Health Care Consultant
Kent Island, Maryland

Sandra B. Martin Whittier, RN, BSN
Director of Nursing
American Home Care Services, Inc.
Salem, Massachusetts

Margaret A. Powers, RN, BSN, MS, CNA
Clinical Director of Surgical/Critical Care Nursing
Greater Baltimore Medical Center
Baltimore, Maryland

Margaret Sharp Woodard, RN, BSN
Nurse Clinician
Home Infusion Therapy Program
Medical College of Virginia Hospitals
Richmond, Virginia

About the Author

T. M. Marrelli received a Bachelor's degree in Nursing from Duke University School of Nursing in Durham, North Carolina and received a Master of Arts degree in Management and Supervision, Health Care Administration, from Central Michigan University. Ms. Marrelli is the author of two other nursing books, also published by Mosby: *Handbook of Home Health Standards and Documentation Guidelines for Reimbursement* and *Nursing Documentation Handbook*.

Ms. Marrelli has extensive experience in hospital, home health, and hospice administration and has worked for the Health Care Financing Administration, where she received the Bureau Director's Citation. Ms. Marrelli is listed in the World Who's Who of Women, 1993/1994. Ms. Marrelli provides consultation services on various aspects of health care, especially the areas of documentation, operations, and management. Correspondence, including feedback about this text, may be directed to the author at Health Care Consulting, Suite 159, 3 Church Circle, Annapolis, MD, 21401.

Preface

When I first became a new manager, no one told me many of the things, that, in retrospect, I needed to know. From the running of successful staff meetings to dealing with hospital administration, I learned to manage by trial and, many times, by error. To ease your journey and to refresh and reinforce management skills you may have already developed is the goal of this book. Staff nurses sometimes receive more extensive orientation and planned educational programs than the managers who supervise them! As managers, we and our staffs deserve better. I hope this book helps fill this gap.

This book is a practical guide to day-to-day operations for nurses who manage people, care plans, or groups of patients. This book is designed to assist nurses recently placed in management positions. It also serves as a refresher for more experienced nurse managers. As hospitals and other patient care settings experience decreasing lengths of stay and increasing patient acuity, the professional nurse must manage more responsibilities in a shorter time frame.

It is unfortunate that some of us have encountered ineffective managers and unproductive or unpleasant management environments. My hope is that this book will help you become a competent, communicative manager and help you take the steps needed to improve your work circumstances, if necessary.

Some important information, usually not included in nursing books, has been incorporated, such as how to market yourself, how to honestly evaluate your own capabilities and needs, and how to manage stress for both you and your staff.

Many of the specific guidelines and descriptions included in the book address nursing management in hospital inpatient settings. However, the general management principles and techniques described can be applied in any nursing care delivery setting, including the increasingly important areas of home care, ambulatory hospice, and long-term care. For example, principles of effective time management and communications are relevant regardless of the particular practice setting. Likewise, hiring and other human resource skills are needed and appropriate to all health settings. Because nursing management of day-to-day operations in homecare and in hospitals differ significantly, I have written Chapter 12 ("The Nurse Manager in Homecare and Hospice"), which describes how to effectively manage day-to-day nursing activities in homecare settings.

Some special features have been included to make this book easy to use. Helpful tips, listed as behavioral strategies, are listed in every chapter. Glossaries to help you more easily understand unfamiliar terms are included for both Chapter 7, "Budgeting Basics" and Chapter 8, "Legal Issues and Risk Management." A summary concludes each chapter. Resources for further professional development, including lists of relevant conferences and certification programs, as well as a list of suggested readings, are provided at the end of the book.

The process of becoming a competent and effective manager is a growth journey, unique to each nurse and to each specific work environment. This book was created to facilitate this process.

T. M. Marrelli, RN, MA

Acknowledgements

I would like to thank the many reviewers and professional associates who listened to more discussions about effective management than they ever cared to hear. Specifically, I want to thank Charles Marrelli, Jane Ostmann, Nina Bell, Jim Snodgrass, Harriet Deutsch, and Bill Glass for their insights and needed humor.

I especially want to thank Darlene Como, Executive Editor, and Brigitte Pocta, Associate Developmental Editor, with Mosby for their support and all their hard work. It is very appreciated.

Contents

5 Day-to-Day Operations, 91

Margaret A. Powers
T. M. Marrelli

6 Effective Time Management and Productivity, 119

T. M. Marrelli

7 Budgeting Basics, 134

Lynda Hilliard

8   Legal Issues and Risk Management, 164

Elizabeth Hogue

9   Quality Assessment and Improvement, 194

T. M. Marrelli

CHAPTER 1

The Nurse Manager Role Today

T. M. Marrelli

Congratulations! Because of your clinical expertise, education, and other valued traits, you were promoted to a management position. Yet the process of becoming an effective manager does not happen overnight. It is a growth process unique to each nurse and specific environment. Whether you are a new manager or a manager new to a facility with a new group, you need to know you are not alone and may need some insights to help you through this period of transition. The people you will be managing are unique and are the most positive part of this position. The manager and staff all work together to meet the organizational goals, as defined in your employer's mission statement and nursing philosophy. Any new role is exciting, but it can also be anxiety producing.

This book was written to help facilitate the process of becoming an effective manager. This book is a guide to day-to-day operations and includes skills and techniques necessary for nurses in management roles. Because of ever increasing opportunities for nurses, proportionately more management roles, expansions of roles, and promotions are available. According to the 1991 nursing compensation survey reported in "Modern Healthcare," raises for managers outpaced raises for staff nursing positions for the second consecutive year. In addition, the average salary for managers rose 13.1%.[1] As hospitals and other patient areas experience decreasing lengths of stay coupled with increased patient acuity and turnover, the professional nurse in a leadership role must manage more responsibilities in a shortened time frame. The learning needs of managers are varied and complex, covering various fields of study. In addition, as health care delivery has changed, so too has the diversity of settings in which nurses manage. Nurses may practice in more than one of the following settings over the course of their careers: hospitals, community health programs, hospices, urgent care centers, outpatient surgical centers, and home health agencies. Other areas include day care programs, office practices, health maintenance organizations (HMOs), preferred provider organizations (PPOs), and other clinical centers.

ROLE TRANSITION

Too often, professional nurses in any health care setting receive little formal management training before becoming part of the management team. It is the nurse's education that ultimately facilitates the role transition to manager. Once a nurse is promoted, it is thought that some skills may have to be changed or even unlearned. The challenge is to provide new managers with the information and skills needed to develop fundamental and successful behaviors and thought processes that effectively contribute to work accomplishment.

Luckily, most new nurse managers bridge parts of this gap using the clinical and educational experiences they bring to the new position. These skills are what nurses do well everyday, including communicating, planning, organizing, prioritizing, and documenting. All are talents that lend themselves well to the new role of nurse manager. Expansion into the nurse manager role is based on management behaviors including planning, organizing, directing, controlling, and evaluating.

The nurse manager's orientation should follow a formal plan. It is important to note that no program, however well thought-out, can address all the issues that will confront the new nurse manager. Some skills fully develop only after a period of time and the integration of knowledge and practice. These good habits become "automatic" only with use.

All change is stressful, even though it may be experienced as good or bad. Some of the most frequently cited causes of stress include vague role descriptions and adapting to what may be perceived as continual change. We know that all nurses experience stress. The new nurse manager has the additional stress of changing roles and integrating oneself into the organization as a manager. It is important at the onset for the new manager to always look for opportunities in every problem.

Example of Position Description for a Nurse Manager

We have all seen the position description for the nurse manager enumerating various responsibilities:

1. The nurse manager is responsible for the staffing, organization, and coordination of patient care 24 hours a day.

2. Develops, administers, and evaluates goals and objectives for the unit.
3. Provides for cost-effective use of human and material resources consistent with goals of cost containment and productivity while providing quality patient care.
4. Participates in the management process.
5. Problem solves.
6. Directs the activities of subordinates.
7. Identifies systems problems.
8. Provides for the continuing education of staff.
9. Develops and evaluates staff.
10. Provides clinical assistance and consultation.
11. Develops, administers, and ensures compliance with policies and procedures and any applicable governmental and accreditation regulations.
12. Assumes other responsibilities as assigned by supervisor.

Reading this list and reflecting on what the nurse manager actually does daily can make the job seem overwhelming. The actual activities may include attending or chairing meetings, evaluating and counseling staff members, assigning or reassigning schedules, and myriad other functions. As we move towards a greater focus on outcome (i.e., a satisfied patient whose needs have been met by discharge), we see why this new role is stressful. It is the nursing staff who comforts and cares for patients 24 hours a day. It is the nursing staff who coordinates all activities related to the patient. These activities are multifaceted and complex and range from clinical tests to therapeutic interventions.

Because of increased specialization of health care providers and complexity of patient problems and associated technology, multiple and varied services are provided to patients. Patients and their families and friends look to the professional nurse for quality care.

Health Care Changes Affecting Nursing Management

Four major factors contribute to the changes that are affecting nursing management.

1. *The current economics of the health care system and utilization management*
   • In response to spiraling health care costs, third-party payers (government, commercial, and business self-insurers) have in-

creased their scrutiny of expensive hospital and other health services. Programs such as utilization review or utilization management have been influential in decreasing lengths of hospital stays.

- Decreased lengths of stay typically cause patients to have acute nursing care needs in a shortened period. The phrase sometimes heard to describe this phenomenon is "quicker and sicker," referring to the patient's status at discharge. Ten years ago the same patient population would have been hospitalized for longer periods. Today much hospital care is provided on an out-patient-only basis.
- Clinical documentation often is the basis on which third-party payers make payment or denial decisions. Nursing documentation often becomes the basis for providing substantiating documentation for a payment or denial determination.

2. *The emphasis on quality in health care*
    - As hospital quality assurance, improvement, and management programs have evolved, patient outcomes are recognized as valid indicators of quality of care.
    - The Joint Commission for the Accreditation of Healthcare Organizations' (JCAHO) new focus on interdisciplinary care creates an atmosphere for the entire health care team to work together to achieve desirable patient outcomes. The JCAHO standards and an indepth discussion of the Quality Assurance/Quality Improvement (QA/QI) processes are discussed in Chapter 10, Quality Assurance and Improvement.

3. *The emphasis on standardization of care, policies, and procedures and the increasing recognition and empowerment of the nursing profession*
    - All patients are entitled to a certain level, or standard, of nursing care. As patients become proactive consumers in the purchase of health care, patient satisfaction with care becomes key to an institution's reputation and ultimate survival. Nurses, because of their healing skills and proficiency and the considerable amount of time they spend with patients and families, are pivotal in achieving patient satisfaction. It is also known that, generally, satisfied patients are less likely to sue. The nurse roles of patient advocate, listener, and teacher have become even more significant in recent years.
    - All professions, including nursing, have recognized standards of care. As society has become more litigious, the professional nurse must be aware of State Nurse Practice Acts and other accepted standards of care. Other standards include hospital poli-

cies and procedures, state and federal regulations, and the published standards of professional nursing organizations. It is important to keep current and informed of professional standards in nursing specialties or other groups and to be aware of the standards of professional nursing practice.

- Health care settings, such as hospitals, also have their own nursing standards of care. Some examples are:
  - Every patient shall have a nursing assessment that is comprehensive, addresses specific patient needs, is performed by a registered nurse at least every _____ hours, and is documented in the patient's record.
  - Discharge planning will begin on admission and includes collaboration with other members of the health team and involves the patient, family, and caregivers.

Through complete and effective documentation, nursing demonstrates that the standard of care has been met.

- There continues to be a great need for qualified nurses in the workplace. Recently the *American Journal of Nursing*[2] stated that the demand for nurses will increase by 38.9% by the end of the century. The U.S. Department of Labor projects that 613,000 new registered nurse (RN) positions will be created during this same time.

4. *The emphasis on effectiveness and efficiency in health care*
  - As health care settings and hospitals continue to streamline, administrative tasks historically performed by nurses are being examined. Repetitive or duplicative activities, as can be found in some documentation systems, are inefficient. Better ways are being explored to meet patient needs while freeing nurses for other important activities.
  - Considering these tumultuous changes in the current health care environment, we see why the nurse manager role is so important today. All these factors create an environment where the nurse has more responsibilities and less time in which to do them. Because of the many tasks that must be undertaken or delegated, flexibility is a necessity for effective nurse managers.

WHAT DOES THE NURSE MANAGER DO?

Core duties that nurse managers assume, regardless of setting, include assignments, delegation, meetings, performance evaluations, budgets, writing and interpersonal skills, and 24-hour accountability for the area. Nurse managers must blend business and clinical skills and perspectives. Because the bulk of the manager's education focused on clinical nursing, it is the business side that usually needs additional educational emphasis. The nurse manager, to be effective, creates an environment that empowers staff to grow professionally. The staff are encouraged to identify problems, recommend and implement solutions, and evaluate outcomes. The staff "own" their issues and work as a group for resolution. Most importantly, the staff achieve patient goals while adhering to policies and the mission statement of the health care setting. The nurse manager is the link between staff and upper management. This role, by definition alone, imparts significant influence and power.

The actual day-to-day operational duties of the nurse manager can be as varied as the practice area of responsibility. In a hospital or a home health agency, for example, the activities are focused on the patient, the consumer of the needed services. The nurse manager, by position and personality, sets the tone for the effective completion of these activities. In patient care settings, the goal of these activities is a satisfied customer. The nurse manager may possess and use the following types of power to achieve this goal:

Coercive power—As implied, this is the power to inflict some type of punishment. This is universally seen as the weakest type of power.
Expert power—The power commanded by special knowledge or competence. This may include degrees, certification, publication, or other skills.
Legitimate power—The power given to exert authority because of a position or title.
Referent power—The personal power of the individual. An example is a person with a motivating personality.
Reward power—The power to bestow or withhold something valued by another person.

The nurse manager's clinical skills will be used in the management role—if only as a resource for staff members (expert power). Some people theorize that a nurse manager, to be effective, must have strong clinical skills. This strong knowledge base may command immediate respect from staff and physicians. Although this may hold true in some clinical areas, it may not be true in all settings.

The new nurse manager has tools available to appear powerful. Initially, the manager's title alone will lend some legitimate power. However, because "testing" by staff is often a part of the transition process, the following descriptions identify how power "looks," or is perceived.

SIX WAYS TO APPEAR MORE POWERFUL

✔ Powerful people usually appear to be calm and unflappable.

✔ Powerful people usually speak less and listen more.

✔ Powerful people exude confidence in themselves and in their problem-solving abilities.

✔ Powerful people are usually optimistic.

✔ Powerful people set appropriate limits for themselves, their resources, and their staff.

✔ Powerful people may not always feel that way, but they have learned to act powerful and know the behaviors and feelings will follow.

THREE WAYS TO ACQUIRE POWER

✔ Ensure that an ongoing educational program is available and includes an orientation program for new staff RNs. Your attendance accomplishes two goals: you learn what new nurses are taught and learn more about the health system or institution.

✔ Participate in educational endeavors, such as pursuing a degree, certification, or learning in another area of interest. Information about certification is addressed in Chapter 13; additional information is listed in the appendix.

✔ Network with other nurse managers on an ongoing basis. This peer support is invaluable for problem solving support and builds morale.

29 BEHAVIORS TO HELP YOU DURING THE TRANSITION

As a new nurse manager it is important that you recognize your own limitations while learning your new role. This can be accomplished initially by the following behaviors:

✔ Recognize and accept that, initially, it is okay to learn, listen, and observe.

✔ Resist the urge to intervene and change how things have been done historically. This means not making big changes initially. Change may be needed, but it may be more successful and acceptable to staff members if their input is sought after you have become the nurse manager in practice and perception. This will also allow for a thorough assessment of the problem and identification of possible solutions and implications.

✔ Remember that the nursing process is an effective tool for problem solving and evaluation.

✔ Use the initial weeks as time to gather data and learn about the organization, daily routines, and your new staff.

✔ Remember that it is okay to NOT have an answer for all problems or issues that staff members may want to lay at your door. Direct the staff, as they are close to the problems and therefore often the best source for effective solutions, to develop possible solutions for problems. This approach empowers the staff by valuing their input and may lead to team problem resolution.

✔ Know that it is okay to ask your staff's input in the decision making process whenever they are affected or know the problem. Let them "own" problems and solutions.

✔ Develop your own management style. You possess unique skills and traits that can be effectively used as a manager.

✔ Know that your unique individual presence will ultimately become your style. Observe managers you respect and add the behaviors you want to emulate to your repertoire. All managers have inherent personality traits. Make the best ones work for you. For example, some managers use humor very effectively. However, this would not work for a manager to whom humor does not come naturally.

✔ Seek ways to understand and motivate your staff. Dale Carnegie is credited with saying that there is only one way to get anybody to do anything; that is by making the other person want to do it. There is no other way. With this statement in mind, a good manager learns what specifically motivates staff members.

✔ Ask for feedback from peer managers or others you trust.

✔ Create an environment of cooperation through your example.

✔ Act and look like a manager. It has been said that perception looks like reality. If you make this leap of faith initially and successfully, so too will others. Observe the behaviors, dress, manners, and people skills of managers and past and present mentors you respect.

✔ Cultivate a positive relationship with your boss. Keep in mind that this important relationship may affect your overall success with the organization in the future.

✔ Communicate clearly, both in writing and in speaking. Communications should be succinct and true. Always validate information before stating facts or committing them to paper.

✔ Practice visualizing yourself as an effective manager. See yourself dealing effectively in a given situation. Practice this by trying it out behaviorally; then evaluate your actions, the process, and the outcome achieved.

✔ Recognize and accept that you cannot have all the right answers and knowledge all the time.

✔ Believe that you are the best person for this job.

✔ Give up on trying to initially address all identified problems.

✔ Remember that, in time, role ambiguity will give way to role definition.

✔ Develop, maintain, and ultimately increase and use your sense of humor. All nurse managers must have a well-developed sense of humor as a stress management tool for self and staff and, where appropriate, for patients, families, and visitors. The inherent healing value of humor is finally being recognized.

✔ Prioritize and think through problems before acting. Some problems will resolve themselves, others may not be yours. Those remaining need to be acted on.

✔ Remember that earning respect and credibility from your staff may take time.

✔ Understand that your staff look to you as role model, teacher, and resource.

✔ Realize that sometimes you need to (diplomatically) rock the boat. Being a successful manager requires taking some risks.

✔ Remember that, while you may not think your boss is always right, he or she is still the boss and as such has an inherent power.

✔ Accept that some of your decisions may not be popular. This does not mean that your decisions are wrong or that you are not a likeable person.

✔ Recognize that during the role transition, one of the most difficult realizations is that you are no longer a staff nurse but a manager. Former peers, now staff members, may no longer confide in you and you may feel isolated. New peer networks and relationships need to be established.

✔ Remember that there is always more to learn.

✔ Realize that your staff is the key to getting all work accomplished.

Assuming the New Role

It is important from the onset that you firmly establish yourself as the new nurse manager. Hold a staff meeting as soon as possible after the announcement of your assumption of the position. Plan a meeting for each shift. For consistency, use the same agenda for all meetings. When in these meetings, keep in mind the "Six Ways to Appear More Powerful" listed on p. 7.

Your First Staff Meeting As New Nurse Manager

The meeting's goals are to formalize your new role with the staff members, introduce yourself, and begin meeting your staff. At this initial meeting:

- Welcome everyone and introduce yourself
- Have everyone introduce themselves
- Speak briefly about your qualifications

An example would be, "As some of you know, I have my BSN and have worked at St. Elsewhere General for 7 years in cardiac rehab. I look forward to the challenge of being the nurse manager of your new cardiac step-down unit and to working with you. Please let me know any recommendations you may have, as I am open to better ways of doing things. Initially, I'll be in orientation and will be scheduling time on all shifts to get to know everyone and the patient routines."

TIPS FOR CONDUCTING INITIAL STAFF MEETINGS

✔ Be aware that staff meetings and their management can be difficult even for experienced nurse managers.

✔ Reassure your staff that you will not be making any changes initially and that you will be observing and speaking to patients and staff members to learn the daily operational routines. This reassurance is needed at this time to decrease staff anxiety about a new manager and more changes.

✔ Share that you will be having similar meetings with the rest of the staff (if that's your plan) and will make rounds on all shifts with team leaders as part of your orientation.

✔ Do say that change is difficult for everyone and you are interested in their input.

✔ Reassure them you will not be changing representatives (again, if true) to the nursing practice council, the product selection committee, or other committees.

✔ Do not be offended if all staff members don't attend. Some staff members may act out or be complacent or appear uninterested. Change is difficult for all!

✔ Keep brief minutes, including attendance, topics discussed, and outcomes accomplished to share with staff members who were not able to attend the meeting.

✔ Always open with a welcome and state how long the meeting will last. Start on time and, when the end of the meeting is near, start wrapping up. An example of a closing statement might be, "We have a few minutes left, we need to come to a decision."

✔ As nurse manager and often chairperson of the meeting, remember to plan for factors such as the logistics of time, place, and dates. Keep in mind also that the best attended and most successful meetings often include food. Some managers have luncheon meetings to capitalize on this fact.

For a more in-depth discussion about conducting or leading meetings, please refer to Chapter 5, "Day-To-Day Operations."

YOUR ORIENTATION

By title you are now a part of the management team. Some power has been transferred to you by your new position and by your knowledge before the promotion. As professionals, all nurses perform some management functions. Staff nurses manage teams of patients, equipment, and clinical environments. They delegate as team leaders and assign duties. The leadership role inherent in RN education moves the nurse to the head of the team. The successful nurse manager integrates these past roles with the knowledge base of sound principles in day-to-day operations. It is these behaviors coupled with learned skills that makes the nurse manager unique.

The new nurse manager has a unique and well-known theory available throughout this transition. The nursing process can be readily applied to management in individual patient care scenarios and in the larger view of the hospital system, which spans multiple departments and services.

AN ORIENTATION CHECKLIST

The following basic information and resources should be readily available to you as a new nurse manager. If not, you may need to tailor an orientation program for yourself with the help of your nursing supervisor:

✔ Typical hours of the nurse managers in the setting

✔ Tour of the facility

✔ The shifts available to staff (e.g., 8, 10, or 12 hours)

✔ Organizational chart

✔ Position description for nurse manager and staff

✔ Facility's policy and procedure manuals

✔ Personnel policy manuals

✔ Information regarding other policies (e.g., if, when, and where smoking is permitted)

✔ Location, hours, and types of material available in staff library

✔ Mentor, peer, or other manager orientation program(s)

✔ Information regarding continuing education and reimbursement policy

✔ Other, based on your specific learning needs

MEETINGS WITH PEER MANAGERS OF OTHER AREAS

As a manager you need to understand the workings and specific functions of areas with which your unit or department frequently interacts. It is also helpful to get to know your peers, the managers of these areas. Setting up a meeting with these managers enables you to gather needed information and begin to network with your peers.

To be effective, a nurse manager needs information about the areas listed in Appendix 1-1.

EIGHT TIPS TO LEARN MORE FROM SCHEDULED ORIENTATION MEETINGS

The following suggestions will help you maximize the value of your peer manager meetings.

✔ See these meetings as informational and networking sessions.

✔ Decide what information you want to learn.

✔ Think about the specific questions you want answered.

✔ From these meetings, consider possible actions to improve operations on the unit.

✔ Ask specific questions.

✔ Write clear, detailed notes for future reference; these notes can also serve as a source of information in the orientation of new nursing staff members.

✔ These meetings should be informational and only for meeting peers; withhold any criticisms at these introductory meetings.

✔ Remember, first impressions are important. Put your best foot forward.

The peer managers you meet at these meetings may become part of your support group at work. They may become friends or important allies who help you achieve your unit's and the organization's goals. They may have interpersonal, budgetary, or other skills you will want to learn.

TAKING TIME TO TAKE STOCK

During your learning and growth period it is appropriate and helpful to review your actions and accomplishments periodically. Questions may include:

- What did I accomplish or learn today?
- What did I learn from my staff, peer managers, and boss?
- On a scale of 1 to 10, how successful was I in achieving the goals I set for today?

- What did I do especially well that makes me feel proud?
- What can I do better the next time?
- What do I need help with and who can I ask for help?
- Did I visualize my success before I acted it out?

Most importantly, recognize that every issue and its resolution adds to your knowledge base of experience and leads to more successes in the future.

IMPORTANT REALIZATIONS

The following realizations may be helpful during your transition to your new nursing management role. Often it takes new nurse managers many months to reach these important and perhaps surprising realizations.

- Resources (financial, personnel, and material) are limited and they will probably become more limited in the future as health care facilities continue to face fiscal constraints.
- There are rarely (if ever) enough hours in the work day.
- One new nurse manager cannot fix all the problems that have plagued a particular unit for years, perhaps even decades.
- People, including your staff, manager, and staff from other departments, will want more from you than you can reasonably give. Learning how and when to say no diplomatically is essential to your health and well being as well as to your success.
- Your health care institution may not adapt well to change.
- There is a "good-old-boy" (or girl) network in many work environments. You may be faced with one at your institution. If you can not or do not want to join it, you will need to learn to work around it. Chances are you will not be able to be effective by ignoring it.
- What the institution or your supervisor says may be different from the behaviors and rules they implement; when this occurs remember that actions speak louder than words.
- You are not responsible for all of the problems at your workplace. Only own and work on those which are truly yours.
- Most nurses and nurse managers are women. If you are a woman, assumptions may be made that you will take care of and fix everything for everyone. It is up to nurse managers to be effective role models and to not reinforce the belief that women are selfless caretakers.

SUMMARY

Although management may have inherent pitfalls, effective nurse managers can make positive, lasting impressions on numerous patients, families, and staff. The new nurse manager may feel isolated and inadequate. Conversely, the successful resolution of problems and the delicate handling of personnel issues leave a feeling of accomplishment like no other. Nurses blend complex healing technology with nurturing care. This combination is why patients and their families marvel at the profession and those skills brought to the bedside.

However, problems are inevitable, and some days the hassles may seem overwhelming. Yet problems present opportunities for personal growth and satisfaction in problem resolution. Use your orientation time to get to know others in your facility and to learn from their experience. They will be glad that someone values their knowledge and expertise.

Transition from staff nurse to the leadership position of nurse manager can be a difficult process. The initial enthusiasm, pride, and fantasies to fix the system must ultimately be tempered with a realistic role identification and realistic goal setting.

REFERENCES

1. Perry L: Nursing supervisors continue to lead climb up the ladder, *Mod Healthcare* p 27, May 27, 1991.

2. NewsCaps: 613,000 new RN jobs projected, *Am J Nurs* 90(1): 74, 1990.

Checklist of Key Information About Important Services and Departments

CHAPLAINCY SERVICES

_____ Types of services (e.g., bereavement, remembrance, worship services, baptisms, other)

_____ Hours the chaplain or other representative chaplaincy staff is available

_____ How a referral is initiated

_____ Other

DATA PROCESSING

_____ Orientation to nursing and other information systems (hardware and software)

_____ Video display terminal (VDT) password and confidentiality safeguards

_____ Management reports and their retrieval

_____ Other

DIETARY OR FOODS SERVICES

_____ Schedule of meal and snack delivery times

_____ Flexibility of menu based on specific patient needs (e.g., kosher, macrobiotic)

_____ Location and hours of restaurants, cafeterias, and snack bars

_____ Staff cafeteria hours

_____ Other

DISCHARGE PLANNING

_____ Resources available to patients, families, and staff

_____ Policy of patients being evaluated on admission

_____ The referral process

_____ The schedule for discharge planning rounds held in the clinical area

_____ Other

FINANCE

_____ How often the unit financial and other utilization reports are generated

_____ Your responsibilities regarding specific reports

_____ The budget processes and timeframes

_____ The process for requesting new capital equipment

_____ Your role in the budget process

_____ The historic supply use baseline for the clinical area

_____ The current occupancy rate

_____ The facility's breakdown of types of payers
_____ Percentage of charity care the facility provides annually and the amount that gets written off
_____ The average length of stay
_____ Other

HUMAN RESOURCES/PERSONNEL

_____ The process of nurse selection
_____ The nurse manager's interview occurs at what point after the nurse recruiter has validated licensure and references
_____ Nurse recruiter responsibilities
_____ Policies and procedures for counseling
_____ Status of union involvement
_____ Overtime and on-call salary guidelines
_____ Availability of a professional nursing pool, either in-house or through nursing agencies on a temporary basis
_____ Actions to take if you believe a nurse is impaired
_____ The standard policy for hiring, evaluation, and termination
_____ Grievance policy and process
_____ Location on the unit of the institution's personnel handbook
_____ Other

LABORATORY SERVICES

_____ Hours of service, pick-up schedule, stat bloods, prn delivery schedule
_____ Find out who is responsible for venipunctures, starting intravenous (IV) solutions, and maintaining IVs and other lines
_____ Other

MEDICAL RECORDS

_____ Policy on patients accessing their clinical charts
_____ Protection of confidentiality if clinical records are data entered or keyed directly into a computerized system
_____ Services and results accessible via the video display terminal (VDT)
_____ Type of medical record system that is in place
_____ Types of charting that are the standard or acceptable
_____ Existence of an institution-wide charting process?
_____ Role of nurses pertaining to documenting in the same clinical note areas as physicians and other professional team members
_____ The program's or hospital's use of problem-oriented medical record (POMR), SOAP, or focus charting
_____ Requirements for computerized documentation in lieu of clinical entries or narrative notes
_____ Other

QUALITY IMPROVEMENT/RISK MANAGEMENT

_____ The roles of these departments in the facility
_____ The process and use of incident reports

_____ When to call the risk manager
_____ Status of studies currently underway (e.g., on patient falls, medication errors, or the use of restraints)
_____ How the nursing manager and staff members receive feedback on the findings
_____ Your areas of responsibilities regarding quality improvement
_____ How nursing integrates with the overall quality improvement process of the hospital
_____ Other

REHABILITATION SERVICES

_____ Services available (e.g., physical, occupational, respiratory therapies and speech-language pathology [SLP] services)
_____ How referrals are initiated
_____ Policy on all CVA patients receiving a swallowing evaluation on admission
_____ Ascertain which department does swallowing evaluations at the institution—occupational therapy (OT) or SLP
_____ Ascertain if the schedules for patient pick-up are posted for the nursing staff
_____ Learn who at the facility does chest PT (e.g., PT, RT, or RN)
_____ Length of time the patient is usually gone from the unit
_____ Accessibility of the charting entries by these professional associates
_____ The schedule for interdisciplinary team meetings
_____ Other

RADIOLOGIC SERVICES

_____ Hours of services
_____ Availability of MRI
_____ Location of services
_____ The process for scheduling and transport of patients
_____ Availability and policy for portable X-ray examinations
_____ Ascertain who holds patients in position for X-ray examinations after hours
_____ Ascertain which X-ray examinations are not done after certain hours
_____ Other

HOME HEALTH CARE

_____ The admission policies
_____ Which types (severity, diagnosis, specialty areas) of patients are appropriate for referral to the program
_____ The geographic boundaries
_____ The referral process
_____ Status of nurse-to-nurse communication for continuity of the plan of care before discharge
_____ Whether the patient meets his or her primary home care nurse, when possible, before discharge
_____ How soon after discharge the patient is assessed in the home setting

_____ Lists of supplies the in-patient nurse should send home with the patient for initial wound or other care

_____ Existence of 24-hour on-call service

_____ How patients are admitted on the weekends

_____ Other services available to support patients and their families at home, such as personal emergency response systems or private duty care

_____ Other areas of expertise offered, such as home IV administration or total parenteral nutrition (TPN)

_____ How the need for services at home is determined and who makes the determination for needed services

_____ How durable medical equipment or other needs are addressed

_____ Status of the agency (e.g., licensed, Medicare certified, and JCAHO or National League for Nursing [NLN] accreditation)

_____ Other

HOSPICE

_____ How a referral is initiated and the admission policies

_____ Where the patient goes if in-patient care is necessary

_____ When the hospice nurse meets the patient and family before hospital discharge for continuity of care

_____ The geographic boundaries

_____ Acceptance of both pediatric and adult patients

_____ The bereavement support process

_____ Support groups for the family

_____ Other

STAFF EDUCATION

_____ The organizational structure for staff development

_____ The scheduled conferences or resources planned for the next two quarters (or other specified time frame)

_____ Availability of clinical preceptors, instructors, or specialists to the staff

_____ Research that is currently occurring in the clinical setting

_____ Ascertain if the orientation program is competency based and how competency is measured

_____ The needs assessment tools currently in use

_____ The mechanism for reevaluation and how often they are reevaluated

_____ Learn what program is currently employed to assist new graduates in their transitions to proficient, professional nurses

_____ The specific resources (e.g., human, fiscal, audiovisual) available to the nurse manager and his or her staff

_____ Ascertain if the manager of staff development is a peer resource for new nurse managers

_____ Ask if there is a peer support program for the staff development team?

_____ Status of JCAHO and/or ANA Nursing Staff Development Standards in the program

_____ The resources available for specialty training (e.g., maternal/child, hospice, home care, operating room, or critical care staff)

_____ Other

Other areas could include housekeeping, facility management, and numerous specialty areas, depending on the size, resources, and structure of the facility.

CHAPTER 2

Management: An Overview

Sandra Martin Whittier

MANAGEMENT: WHAT IS IT?

New nurse managers are experienced at nursing but new to management. Initially, the new manager can focus on the following principles, outlined by McGregor[1]:

- Subordinates' need for security
- An atmosphere of approval
- Consistent discipline
- Knowledge of hospital rules, regulations, and procedures
- Knowledge of change in advance
- Knowledge of hospital policy and management philosophy

The purpose of organization will enlighten the manager as to the management philosophy and reporting mechanisms of the agency or hospital. Departmental goals, documentation procedures, use of the nursing process, and any theoretical basis used for practice guidelines are communicated via the direct supervisor of the new manager.

Managers must have a clear understanding of the mission of the agency or organization and be able to communicate to staff in ways that promote understanding and adoption of that mission. Abilities and skills necessary for such communication are listed in the accompanying box.

WHAT IS LEADERSHIP?

Nurse managers are chosen for their leadership ability and demonstrated clinical competence. Earlier in their careers, they performed well when "in charge," were complimented by staff or supervisors, and began to see themselves differently. At some point they discov-

ABILITIES AND SKILLS NEEDED BY NEW NURSE MANAGERS

ABILITIES
- Influence workers to believe in themselves
- Develop individual staff strengths
- Create a desire for excellence and loyalty
- Work with staff behaviorally to improve weaknesses
- Provide challenges in the context of a busy day
- Evaluate performance constructively
- Mentor both staff members who display leadership characteristics and those who require coaching
- Communicate with their managers and staff to outline responsibilities and decision making
- Lead by example
- Demonstrate knowledge of human behavior and its motivation
- Motivate staff members to work together
- Administer departmental budgets
- Communicate clearly and nonjudgmentally
- Be consistent
- Be flexible
- Take risks

SKILLS
- Demonstrate clinical excellence
- Make effective decisions
- Evaluate the clinical knowledge and skills of individual staff members to match staff to patients
- Implement reasonable staffing schedules on a timely basis
- Have vision to plan for next week or month while getting through today
- Create a stimulating environment that encourages staff autonomy
- Develop short- and long-term goals with your staff's input
- Acknowledge that staff members need to ventilate emotions and allow this in the proper setting
- Display commitment
- Build effective work groups
- Make performance evaluations a positive experience
- Empower your staff
- Provide positive reinforcement—often and loudly
- Choose not to be intimidated by a "potential" or "defacto" manager
- Encourage professional growth of staff by exposure to clinical seminars or conferences

ered their innate leadership skills, a foundation on which to build and add new skills.

Leadership is the key to management. Bethel[2] describes 12 qualities of leadership. According to Bethel, a leader:

1. Has a mission that matters
2. Is a big thinker
3. Has high ethics
4. Masters change
5. Is sensitive
6. Is a risk taker
7. Is a decision maker
8. Uses power wisely
9. Communicates effectively
10. Is courageous
11. Is a team builder
12. Is committed

Leading is guiding and directing the skills of others toward positive outcomes. Leaders must continually examine and develop their own skills to remain confident in their abilities.

Just as confidence and enthusiasm are contagious, insecurity can be sensed and targeted by some staff. Leaders must be perceptive and have acute powers of observation when evaluating the group's cohesiveness. Divisive staff members challenge the manager to keep strengthening and reevaluating leadership skills. Leadership is essential to orderly direction in supporting the staff in quality patient care.

Types of Leaders

Excellent nursing leadership requires being action-, results-, or outcome-oriented.[3] Leading by example, being available to staff when needed, constantly sharpening skills, and having an earnest understanding of staff concerns are important to creating loyalty and respect between staff members and manager. Leaders are problem-solvers who do not see a problem as an obstacle to *overcome* but as a puzzle requiring thought to *solve.*

Two leadership concepts, as defined by Burns,[4] can assist the new manager to establish a style of leading. A transformational leader has a vision that, when shared with the staff, creates motivation for working to accomplish the goal. A transformational leader is dynamic, can see the end result, and can incorporate staff input, thereby illustrating staff creativity. Once staff members see that their suggestions have value, more suggestions will follow, and they will begin to originate their own solutions to other problems.

In contrast, transactional leaders have little vision and are more skilled at managing day-to-day tasks. Transactional leadership concepts can be used as an adjunct to the transformational style, but they may be outdated as a primary leadership style. The transformational leader is described as being committed and having a vision of what can be accomplished. Also, when the leader communicates the vision, the leader empowers staff members to achieve their potential. The transformational leader gives responsibility to employees at all levels to make the most of their talents. The transformational leader encourages learning, exploration, and creativity. Staff members know what needs to be done and believe in the vision, so all accomplish more. This is especially helpful in times of declining resources.[5]

THE MANAGEMENT ENVIRONMENT

All nurse managers face many economic and professional influences that affect their work environment. Some of the most important contemporary influences are listed below.

Economic issues

- Increases in number of patients without health insurance coverage
- More acutely ill patients seeking medical/surgical care
- More pressure for staff members to work as more family members lose jobs in the current economic climate
- Third-party–payor restrictions on care allowed
- Third-party payor's increased expectation of patient participation in care

Professional issues

- AIDS and other infection care
- Value clarification
- Nursing shortage
- Effect of fiscal reductions on ancillary services' staffing levels
- Rotation and weekend work, overtime requests
- "Quicker and sicker" syndrome causing the staff to respond by "doing the best they can"

- Medical/nursing relationships may not be collaborative
- Professional development/continuing education
- Challenges to authority
- Ethics in management of decreasing resources

THE GROWTH OF A NEW MANAGER

Some new managers are fortunate enough to have worked for nurse managers who taught administrative as well as clinical skills. Those without this previous training will have to successfully develop these new skills.

Nurse managers report to managers themselves. Depending on the agency or organization, nurse managers are also influenced by layers of management and agendas, whose downward influence can determine a new manager's effectiveness and longevity. Good managers support, as well as develop, new managers and potential new managers.

Nursing management skills are vital to nursing's continued growth. Adverse economic and professional influences compound the difficulties seen by staff members as deterrents to managerial aspirations. The future of nursing management depends on the growth and positive leadership of staff. Nurse managers foster the development of future nurse managers by:

- Being managerially self-aware
- Nurturing the staff's clinical and leadership potential
- Leading by example
- Demystifying managerial concepts with the staff to increase mutual understanding
- Mentoring other nurses

As resources decrease and work stressors increase, nurse managers must use their individual strengths to promote loyalty in an atmosphere of trust. Creating a stable environment that promotes professional growth, excellence in patient care, and individual problem-solving and goal setting is the role of the nurse manager.

The importance of effective nursing management cannot be underestimated. New managers need guidelines and mentoring, especially through the classic management dilemmas, such as poor work performance or dealing with disruptive staff. Without appropriate nursing direction, new managers will become discouraged and either return to patient care or leave nursing entirely. Nursing cannot afford to lose these potential managers who could have been effective leaders but who never fulfilled the manager role.

STYLES OF MANAGEMENT

Choosing one management style does not allow the nurse manager the flexibility required to meet her own needs or those of the staff. New managers will want to select a style that is satisfying and productive while continuously being developed.

MANAGEMENT STYLES

Research and development to design strategies for managerial use have defined four management styles:

✔ Autocratic

✔ Laissez-faire

✔ Democratic

✔ Participative

✔ *Autocratic managers*
  - Do not delegate
  - Make all decisions
  - Have little or no use for staff input
  - Uses authority to accomplish goals
  - Foster reliance on manager

✔ *Laissez-faire managers*
  - Provide little direction
  - Perform without structure or organization
  - Do not provide guidance
  - Do not foster group cohesion
  - Abdicate decision-making

✔ *Democratic managers*
  - Initiate staff participation
  - Delegate with the purpose of staff development
  - Encourage staff toward goal setting
  - Allow individuals a degree of control
  - Provide frequent positive feedback

✔ *Participative managers*
- Make final decisions, but include staff input
- Negotiate as well as direct
- Enlist staff suggestions
- Provide staff members with opportunities to develop their careers
- Transcend the manager-staff gap

All new managers may incorporate the positive and negative aspects of their own previous managers. Many managers can be categorized based on the management style characteristics they display. It is important to note that staff members also function at varying levels, depending on their former nurse managers.

The tasks of the area, unit, or organization must be reviewed when considering management styles. For example, as a new manager of a critical care unit, the immediacy of response to life-threatening events may require some autocracy in management. Imperative to management style development is the assessment of individual nurses' strengths and weaknesses. The same new critical care manager may have a disproportionate amount of new staff who require more supervision. Therefore a critique of staff performance can be a guide on which to base managerial style selection. In addition, the level of autonomy or professionalism in your staff affects the choice of leadership style.

The concept of situational leadership can be used when considering which management style a group requires. All staff members and managers have various facets that influence their adaptability to change, new direction, or new management. Each staff member and manager has strengths that rise to the surface, often based on clinical experience and problem solving attributes, and these qualities can be matched by the manager to foster growth in other staff members who need improvement in these areas.

To adapt leadership to the situation, the workers' needs, the leader's abilities, and the methods chosen to direct or supervise should be chosen based on whether the required tasks are clear-cut or ambiguous, whether staff members desire structure or independence, and whether the leader is a skilled group worker or an autocrat.[6] Autocracy has its place at times, but no manager of the nineties can use autocracy as a prominent style. Assertiveness of individuals, disappearance of the handmaiden concept of nursing, and changing medical/nursing relationships prohibit managers from directing without staff participation.

Management philosophies focus on the manager's ability to attain cost-effective and productive quality results. Therefore a laissez-faire style, with its lack of focus and direction, is not a useful style for the new nurse manager to develop. This is true in any nursing setting, where the new nurse manager must by her presence and personality lead the staff to work toward development of their potential.

The new nurse manager must have a working knowledge of all leadership styles for use in multiple situations. Communication with confidence is crucial when incorporating a style into the nurse manager's daily repertoire. Consistent reactions by the manager will help staff members adopt an example of a style to use themselves.

Autocratic and laissez-faire styles are extremes in management styles, the former manager making all decisions without staff input, and the latter being unable to make swift and correct decisions. More balanced styles are democratic and participative. These styles allow the manager to develop staff members to a degree that they are often asked, and feel comfortable giving, their opinions for problem solving. Short- or long-term goals generated by the staff are more likely to be successfully achieved when the manager leads democratically. Staff members led by a democratic leader who takes and uses their advice project a feeling of being part of an effective group process. A leader's use of a democratic style in management will not stifle or stagnate the staff. A true leader may find a few specific uses for the autocratic rule, but she will generally depend on democratic and participatory leadership styles. The last two styles promote in staff members their ability and confidence to identify problems and solve them while evaluating effects of both solutions and processes.

Participatory leadership varies from the democratic style of management in several ways. This leader presents the identified problem with potential solutions. Staff input is then invited, but the manager may ultimately decide on the specific implementation. Participatory leadership has its drawbacks. By creating an illusion of participation by soliciting feedback, but then not using the staff suggestions, the nurse manager may unknowingly be sabotaging future efforts to promote participation. Positive aspects of participatory management involve the commitment of sharing authority and responsibility throughout an agency or organization. This is most effectively ensured when the entire organization values participatory management as their philosophy.

Participatory leadership creates a dependency on the leader to identify problems, unlike the democratic style, which encourages staff to initiate and develop ideas. An illustration of the various styles in response to a familiar scene might be:

The autocratic leader—"I have completed the schedule for the holidays, using the policy of staff members working every other holiday. There will be no switching of time among staff members."

The laissez-faire leader—"The holiday schedule is completed by the scheduling office; I can't think of a better way to do it."

The democratic leader—"Mary has an idea to present at the staff meeting about coverage for the upcoming holidays."

The participatory leader—"We will have a staff meeting and complete the holiday schedule as a group."

This choice of leadership styles can be pivotal in being an effective nurse manager. It is important to be aware that staff members will respond negatively to styles and responses that are not consistent. Conversely, even when managers give predictable responses, the staff is at least aware of managerial expectations in given circumstances. The test of managerial success in nursing is successfully developing a comfortable and consistent management style that facilitates growth and satisfaction for both the manager and the staff.

The new manager, while studying management styles, may want to try out her initial responses to employees' performance and apply them to a behavior scale to characterize the style that surfaces. Several tools are available that categorize a manager's responses to the appropriate management style, such as Hersey and Blanchard[7] and Fiedler.[8] One classic example is Tannenbaum and Schmidt's continuum of behavior (Figure 2-1).[9]

Figure 2-1 enables the new manager to problem solve when dealing with various prospective solutions to practical situations. Making use of her knowledge of individual staff members and their needs, as well as her own, the new manager can anticipate new problems while solving others and analyze her own behavior at the same time. The new manager must have enough personal confidence to allow new and seasoned nurses to flourish without feeling that her power or knowledge is usurped or threatened. Nurse managers cannot control the environment by their presence alone and must be able to take a vacation with confidence that daily activities will continue

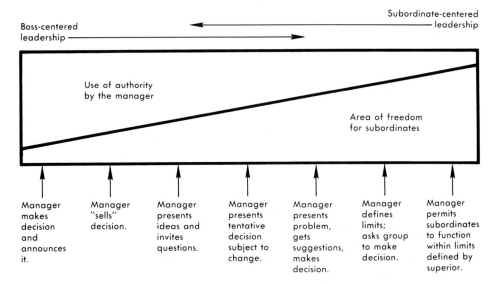

Boss-centered
leadership

Subordinate-centered
leadership

Use of authority
by the manager

Area of freedom
for subordinates

| Manager makes decision and announces it. | Manager "sells" decision. | Manager presents ideas and invites questions. | Manager presents tentative decision subject to change. | Manager presents problem, gets suggestions, makes decision. | Manager defines limits; asks group to make decision. | Manager permits subordinates to function within limits defined by superior. |

FIG. 2-1   Continuum of leadership behavior and participation. (From Tannebaum R, Schmidt WH: How to choose a leadership pattern, *Harvard Bus Rev* 51:164, 1973.)

smoothly. A key sign of a good nurse manager is that the staff functions well whether or not the manager is present.

COMMUNICATION (REGARDLESS OF MANAGEMENT STYLE)

Communication, negotiation, the ability to understand the political process and economics, sensitivity to organizational process, knowledge of how to form alliances, critical thinking, and the ability to construct a solid case for a point of view are some of the skills nurse managers need.[10] Nurse managers can evaluate their communication skills by observing staff response when information is presented. An important aspect of communication is perception. One cannot assume that the staff will always understand and follow through with the agenda communicated by the manager. Verbal communication should be followed up by written, when appropriate. Written staff meeting minutes dispensed to all staff members unable to attend deflects the excuse, "No one ever told me." Clear communication leaves no room for conjecture, and all have an understanding of the material presented. With some staff members, this may require that the nurse manager request immediate feedback to validate the communication.

Two other aspects of communication vital for the new nurse

manager are (1) negotiation and (2) the effective use of positive feedback. Negotiation can be useful as a tool to persuade even the most resistant staff member trying to exercise his or her power, which is a problem situation, against the new manager. The new manager should assess whether this forcefulness results from insecurity of the staff person before using negotiation as a management tool. As an example, suppose a length of time has passed between managers, and this staff nurse has risen to a power position among the staff. This nurse probably needs some time to adjust to changing roles within the group. That power of the "de facto" leader can also be used to enable the staff as the new manager establishes her role.

If the new manager has evaluated the behavior and identifies it as insecurity, positive feedback may dispel any challenges to the manager's power. Positive feedback can be an icebreaker and is always necessary. It can include any praise for any job well done:

- Strong assessment skills
- Handling of an emergency
- Working extra hours
- Support during change
- Support of another staff member—either emotional or physical
- Handling a heavy assignment
- Early detection of clinical signs requiring treatment
- Working together as a team
- Dealing with difficult physicians
- Leadership skills demonstrated by staff
- Dealing with supervisors

This list is by no means complete; please think of your own positive feedback and use it. At the end of each day, some managers thank staff members. Others get in the good habit of giving positive feedback daily. These are not empty words; they contribute positively to staff autonomy and self-esteem. For an in-depth discussion on communication, please see Chapter 4, Communications.

Positive and negative feedback, negotiation, communication skills, and choice of leadership style are the responsibility of new nurse managers. The methodical evaluation, choice, and development of managerial style and characteristics is never time wasted. It is easier for the manager and the staff as a group when the manager selects and implements a style that matches the manager's best skills and begins the process of fostering growth and unity among staff. The long-term effectiveness and excellence with which the organizational goals are attained is worth the effort because then patients' needs are met and professional nursing careers are fulfilled.

THE NURSING PROCESS

Nursing management involves both nursing and management theories. Nursing theories abound and must be studied at greater length than is possible here. Nursing theory can lay the groundwork for nursing standards in any specialty. For instance, Orem's self-care theory[11] is adaptable to community health. Orem's emphasis is on health promotion and states that health information given to the consumer causes change in behaviors that are deemed unhealthy, which is also the basis of community health nursing. Behavior change used as a demonstrated patient outcome can then be formulated into nursing standards of care. Nursing theory can be used when updating or creating nursing standards.

Regulations are promulgated by federal and state agencies or accreditation organizations such as JCAHO. A heightened emphasis is on consumer rights for patients, expected outcomes, and goal achievement. The ongoing review of standards is a part of the responsibility of the nurse manager.

The new manager can use another theory that is very familiar when she is called on to problem-solve, evaluate nursing compliance to standards, or assess quality assurance and quality improvement processes.

Remember the nursing process
Assessment
Planning
Implementation
Evaluation

The nursing process helps the manager track or organize any issue objectively. Once potential solutions are identified, they can be categorized, studied, and, when managers are democratic or participatory in management style, shared with staff for their input and ideas. The manager comes up with an implementation time frame. Once the time frame is met, the evaluation portion is next. The evaluation must continue to remain objective. Thus the cycle is complete, and the next problem or issue can be confronted. The nursing process is one tool managers can use among other nursing and management theories.

WRITTEN RECORDS

The dynamic aspect of the manager role entails that even when you are planning for future needs, the staff's past cannot be forgotten. This historical overview is sometimes helpful to new managers. The long, sometimes tedious process of change and growth must be documented accurately to ensure that the process was true to objectives. A dependable method, which is needed when the manager must provide facts to defend positions, is written communication. Written communication, as an adjunct to the spoken word, can be difficult to incorporate into a busy day, but it is essential that the new nurse manager do so. The practice of committing to memory observations about behavior, good or bad, without actual notations is no longer feasible and is not responsible to the staff. Those guiding new managers must foster the use of anecdotal recording on a daily basis as a management tool and assist new managers to develop strategies to meet this goal.

During meetings with the staff on a group or individual basis, the discussion should be summarized orally and then the plan of action summarized in writing. Short notes kept on the staff's performance can make evaluation time objective and full of examples, positive and negative, on which manager and staff goals are designed. All that must be noted are (1) the topics of discussion and (2) the outcomes or goals for either or both parties. Then the next meeting will first address the progress or steps being taken to meet the goals.

A manager owes the staff a meaningful performance evaluation, citing examples of behavior being reviewed. This helps the manager be more realistic and fair, without being influenced by personality or popularity attributes. Some incidents will be remembered without hesitation; times of high emotion and tragedy, personal losses, and the legions of patients for whose lives the staff fought are emblazoned on everyone's mind. Time passes quickly between events nurses remember, so notation of regular daily activity is a management obligation.

A new manager should begin by writing thoughts when evaluating the staff's performance of patient care, keeping in mind the objectives of the organization. Such documentation can be helpful in other situations; for example, the new manager might record that the staff needs more equipment or training, listing specific examples. She could then discuss this subject with her manager. The documentation then makes important information quickly available when needed. The ability to rapidly provide specific rationales supporting the manager's point is a key to the manager's credibility and ultimate effectiveness.

NURSING MANAGEMENT BY OBJECTIVES

Anecdotal comments and their use as a daily chronicle is beneficial as practice for working with management by objectives (MBO). These anecdotal notes reduce assumption and provide a foundation for evaluating staff performance. MBO for nurses uses the setting and meeting of goals, usually behavioral, that cause improvement in patient care and professional attitude. MBO causes one to strive to attain further goals within a specific period, goals designed at the individual's pace. The use of MBO provides focus and direction to managerial and institutional goals. An objective of a new manager might be, "Evaluate all RNs by observation of their work and documentation, among other factors, and conduct a personal review with each RN by June 30." This objective is measurable and has a specific time frame. Anecdotal documentation assists the manager in meeting this goal. Using MBO is for managers who want to create a new environment for progress and quality patient care. For the benefit of the new manager, MBO can be practiced whether or not the organization promotes it. Once the principles are understood, MBO can help in many ways as a step towards achievement of goals in any organization.

MBO identifies where you fit in, organizationally or within the smaller group you manage. Expectations are put out for discussion and direction for the manager and her group or the manager's meeting with the nursing executive. Clear expectations leave little room for misunderstanding, and individuals must improve or restate their objectives. The staff who do their best identify those who are not effective.

Observation of staff performance, evaluation of written documentation, patient satisfaction surveys, and manager and staff position descriptions can be steps toward identifying realistic goals. Another example of an objective might be—by June 30, 1993, the nurse manager will:

1. Set up June—December in-service topics as prioritized by staff.
2. Accomplish all staff performance evaluations by a specified deadline.
3. Perform documentation reviews in view of agency/institutional standards.

4. Evaluate staffing patterns and rotate once to each shift every ____.
5. Schedule all registered nurses to have a minimum of one week in charge every____.

All objectives must:

- Have a specific time frame
- Be behaviorally stated
- Be objectively evaluated
- Identify positive rather than negative outcomes

MBO CHARACTERISTICS

✔ Sets limits on the time for behavior to change

✔ Uses negotiation

✔ Is effective by making the point cumulatively

✔ Is a clear and concise form of communication

✔ Controls change

✔ Can be used by any level of staff

✔ Varies from the global to very specific

✔ Documents problems beyond the manager's control

✔ Aids analytical thinking

✔ Encourages staff development

✔ Improves skill in planning

Practice of MBO is advantageous to the new manager. Much new information can be categorized and relegated to a step outlined in an objective. This allows the new manager to spend time prioritizing where attention is required first. MBO also lends the novice manager more objectivity, rather than "gut feelings" when learning and being challenged. For example, specific effects on the group by a staff member's tardiness can have extensive ramifications. The nurse manager, on identifying this problem, may create this objective—by Friday:

- Schedule and hold an individual meeting with the tardy staff member.
- Negotiate a contract to stop tardiness. Check personnel policies and procedures manual and staff member's file to assess need for verbal warning.
- List specific tasks done by others, in place of tardy nurse, and any other outcomes of the behavior (e.g., second report).

The new manager will be reacting in the same manner with all the staff using this method. Consistent behavior toward all staff members sends the message that criticism is constructive and fair. The manager's attitude should be positive as much as possible.

Time can thus be spent on unit issues, improving quality as well as improving the staff's enjoyment of their work. Nurses can use objectives to require staff development in meeting individual and group goals. MBO encourages forward thinking by its use of setting objectives for the future.

The nurse manager can also use MBO to guide the staff toward the larger, organizational targets. Dates of accomplishing objectives must be flexible, without negating the use of this tool. Thinking forward using goal setting fosters continued personal growth and open communication.

MBO can be adapted to any work situation and, when gradually introduced, can be a positive growth experience for all. Control of growth by the staff can relieve some of the stressors of nursing in the 1990s. MBO for managers is an adjunct to improving:

- Interviewing
- Negotiating
- Delegating (and then leaving them alone!)
- Sharing power/authority
- Performance evaluation
- Managerial growth
- Development of leadership qualities and management style
- Budgetary responsibilities
- Problem solving
- Building of credibility consistently
- Decision making
- Listening

MANAGEMENT THEORIES

Management philosophy has as many facets as there are organizations. Management philosophy starts with the top level in any organization. Therefore, when the chief executive officer changes, (1) the philosophy may change, and (2) the philosophy of the management team is reassessed.

A review of the levels of management may either confirm or deny the top management's commitment to promote decentralization and manager growth. A new manager in any organization should explore the specific philosophy of the new setting.

QUESTIONS FOR NEW MANAGERS TO ASK

✔ Does this agency hire and promote from within?

✔ Do staff members show job longevity and commitment?

✔ Does management sponsor employee activities that foster effective team building?

✔ Do managers confer with other department heads independently or does everything go through the manager of each department head?

✔ Does this agency promote community activities?

The answers to these questions can give important information about the true organizational philosophy. The management philosophies X and Y, set forth by McGregor,[12] can be summarized as follows:

Theory X—The average human being has an inherent dislike of work and will avoid work where possible. This causes the need for direction and control in employee management.

Theory Y—Physical and mental effort is as natural as play or rest. If employees are committed to organizational objectives, they will be self-directed and need fewer controls.

The organizational controls may be difficult to separate from various regulatory requirements. Some controls instituted and supported are deleterious to recruitment and retention in nursing.[13] The hospital organizational structure and its adherence to tradition is one reason for a decrease in power and decision-making for nurses and an important reason for nursing turnover.

A new management philosophy emerging involves Japanese principles. This approach encourages group participation and, in fact, makes decisions via consensus. This seems an effective way to include nursing, rather than nursing having to demand inclusion, as a voice in the policy-making process, which is often controlled by physicians and administration. It will be interesting to see if this Japanese management philosophy affects nursing in the 1990s.

What the Japanese philosophy expounds is value in the realms of quality, creativity, and commitment. The use of group efforts (called *quality circles*) toward setting objectives to meet stated goals unites the staff to work together. The Japanese philosophy harnesses the ideas that effective staff teams can and will create. It causes the staff to commit to reaching stated and clearly defined goals. This philosophy extols:

- Higher nursing retention rates
- Increased productivity
- Less litigation for malpractice
- Collective decision making
- Staff responsibility
- Stimulation and recognition of staff creativity
- Open communication
- Skill sharing
- Managerial credibility

The steps necessary when initially developing a less authoritarian leadership style or first using Japanese quality circles to stimulate problem-solving can be daunting to the new nurse manager. The nurse manager must be a role model and catalyst and provide an atmosphere of open and honest discussion. Dialogue can cause positive behavior change that improves the level of service and positive patient outcomes. Whichever mechanism is chosen, whether Japanese or traditional American, the managerial philosophies are simply different methods with the same goals. All new nurse managers want to cultivate an environment that encourages unity and excellence in patient care delivery.

Management philosophy ultimately determines the growth and level of fulfillment of the workers. Guidance and direction is provided by the administration to its managers while allowing them the responsibility of decision making and control. Managers work best when they are able to develop staff in a consistent and supportive manner and enjoy the same handling from their own superiors. The management team works most effectively when the environment is collegial, respectful, and nurturing. New managers should elicit advice about the level of support and managerial development systems from both peers and bosses. Gradually increasing responsibility while new managers expand their skills and are groomed in the management philosophy generates strong, decisive, and successful managers. The new nurse manager provides leadership to the staff while learning administrative skills. Past experiences influence practice and behavior in the developing nurse manager.

An immediate source of information and guidance for the new nurse manager is her supervisor. Initially, the new nurse manager should expect frequent meetings, weekly perhaps, and should use this time with her boss wisely. Assessments of staff abilities and needs made by the new nurse manager can be reviewed with the supervisor, with problems and solutions identified. Explanation of channels of communication, rules, and etiquette expected of administration may be covered.

All nurses have role models they chose to emulate during their careers. When these relationships evolve into a mentor-student mode, they are a source of personal and professional support and satisfaction. "Nurse executives need to take every opportunity to place themselves in a mentoring role for nurse managers. Reviewing institutional goals and objectives with nurse managers assists them in creating and identifying a vision for future health care practice environments."[14]

The new nurse manager should evaluate the level of support available from administration. Observing discussions and reactions of the upper management with their managers and peers can give the new nurse manager insight into the hierarchy of the organization. The new manager determines whether the organizational philosophy is compatible with her own values. Ideally, the manager feels wanted, being part of an organization that historically promotes from within and rewards the progress and development of employees.

New nurse managers are thrust into a fast-paced job and so must rapidly determine how much authority is part of the position. If too many decisions are made above the nurse manager's level, she may feel stifled. The nurse manager must then decide whether the organizational goals permit some control and thus make the situation workable, or whether it would be better to move on to a new professional experience.

More often, nurse managers are allowed flexibility in such key tasks as hiring and scheduling. Building on these tools, new nurse managers develop their own style of leadership within the management group.

The nurse manager should strive for certain outcomes in her new role. As the new nurse manager tries to achieve these outcomes, she will develop an ability to analyze the power structure of the organization. The box on pg. 42 lists role outcomes.

ORGANIZATIONAL CHART

Each organization has a formal and an informal communication system and a chain of command that reflects the manager's base of power. Unofficial personal relationships may command more authority than the organizational chart structure, and all new managers should ascertain allies and adversaries. This will take longer for new managers who have also just joined an organization but can also create an opportunity for improved communication among managers and administration. The middle manager is working from both sides, between staff and upper management and, as such, is vital to any organization.

Concepts to evaluate when beginning as a nurse manager are, as noted by Gillies[5]:

- Role
- Power
- Status
- Authority
- Centrality
- Communication

Studying these aspects of agency hierarchy and using communication to validate perceptions is an important exercise for new managers.

There will be occasions that test new managers. This is particularly true when management delivers an edict to the new nurse manager that is contrary to her principles. There are no rules as to which side wins, and this situation can cause both personal and professional stress. Sometimes the new nurse manager's loyalties will be with staff and in conflict with administration or vice-versa, and managers need to know with whom conversation is confidential. New managers need to have a sounding board to assist in formulating answers, especially when directives appear to be unfair to staff.

NEW NURSE MANAGER ROLE OUTCOMES

POSTENTREPRENEURIAL STYLE

The ability to relinquish bureaucratic styles of leadership; more employee-centered with core characteristics of innovation, efficiency, and reward of outcomes; authority derived from expertise and experimentation

EMPOWERMENT

Ability to empower self and staff for quality patient outcomes; ability to influence organizational policy development as related to patient care

VISION

Ability to foresee the growth and development of nursing and managerial practice and strategically plan to assist these processes

ENHANCEMENT OF IMAGE

Ability to identify self as a professional nurse and manager, perceiving self as a leader and enhancing the profession of nursing in the community and organization

FLEXIBILITY

Ability to adapt to turbulence in the organization and practice environment; ability to assess outcomes; ability to design better and newer processes in patient care and management to achieve quality service

CLINICAL EXPERTISE

Ability to identify with those who are managed; staying close to the client and the practice environment to manage the delivery of health care effectively

ANALYTICAL THINKING

Ability to problem solve effectively using logic and decision support systems and models; ability to conduct research in nursing management

LEADERSHIP ROLE IDENTITY

Ability to see self as a leader, mentor, and nurse or patient advocate; ability to assist in meeting institutional goals and objectives through effective performance; ability to get things accomplished

AUTONOMY

Ability to practice nursing and management in a highly decentralized environment without alienation of executive leadership

MASTER CHANGE

Ability to identify, cope with, introduce, and assimilate change successfully in the practice environment

Flarey DL: Redesigning management roles, *J Nurs Adm* 21:44, 1991.

The level of decentralization present in the management structure determines the autonomy allowed. Decentralization permits control or delegation by the nurse manager and the chance to develop and empower the staff. Decentralization promotes manager-manager communications and meetings and avails the nurse manager to other nurse managers or committee chairs of quality assurance, utilization review, continuing education and infection control. Acknowledgement that highly educated or knowledgeable workers can evaluate, design, and implement the complex care required by nurses can be the attitude of an effective decentralized nursing department. Committee memberships add further to the amount of opinions generated and policies implemented on various issues that help establish management styles.

As a middle manager in nursing, the novice needs patience, advice, and a confidante with whom to debate strategy and concerns, pros and cons. Whether or not the manager's supervisor becomes the resource, that relationship is important to cultivate as well. Sometimes staff members become important as allies to the nurse manager. Their support during day-to-day operations and in crises is the real concern of the nurse manager. The manager acts as a filter through which administrative goals are communicated to staff and change directed. As it is possible to change a dressing differently, still using aseptic principles, the nurse manager can divert information not necessary for staff to know and still communicate necessary policy. Many times rationale is explained when change occurs. Administrative policies can be explained and practiced within the style of the nurse manager. As long as organizational principles are maintained, implementation can be staged by the manager.

Through autonomy, independence, and decentralization comes accountability and performance. Efforts at group cohesion and quality must be a result of the manager's ability to motivate and develop staff that is fulfilled and productive. Survival in middle management means success, with respect from both upper management and subordinate staff.

MENTORING

A mentor is someone with whom you can discuss all manner of aspects of management. Mentors usually have similar values, goals, and personalities. The mentor acts as a nurturer who can listen and guide you through dilemmas, each encounter ultimately requiring less input from the mentor. The mentor can lead you by introducing

---

WHAT MENTORS PROVIDE

Guidance dealing with employee behavior problems
Help in developing management style
Coaching
Gradual increase in responsibilities
Nonjudgmental criticism
Encouragement
Teaching of new skills
Desire to further education

---

other personnel who can be resources for you. Mentors act on a personal level, in addition to their career development role.

The mentor must be wise enough to remain loyal through all phases of the new manager's growth. Mistakes may happen and poor judgement be used, and emotional responses must be supported while gently pointing out more positive methods. This could include how to handle administrative edicts with which the new manager strongly disagrees. The capacity to have honest discussions without consequences can be enriching. Principles formed in these early stages of a career will be carried forward, regardless of the work situation, to future professional roles.

The relationship of mentor-protégée can be mutually satisfying. A mentor must be chosen wisely, with a matching of goals, leadership qualities, and personal styles as the foundation. Seeking role models may be a stepping stone toward forming a mentor-protégée relationship. As the novice accumulates experiences, the mentor is also energized. The mentor enjoys a rejuvenation and feeling of purpose.

The mentor may not be a part of the organization of the new manager. When this occurs, the telephone is the usual form of communication. Occasionally, the pair are employed at the same setting and the mentor can observe the management style developing in the new manager.

The mentor relationship has a quality that can expand in times of frustration, change, or self-doubt. During periods of relative stability, the mentor may be needed less. This relationship may last many years and through career changes by either party. The trust developed between the mentor and the new manager will be transferred to other professional relationships and may create a desire in the young manager to become a mentor to other nurses. The nursing environment is greatly improved when nurses provide each other with trust and respect, most especially initially in new management careers.

Mentors and role models are both positive methods that influence, occasionally by their absence, the development of leadership skills in novice nurses. A role model is someone admired by others for their skills and character. A role model is revered, possibly from afar without personal commitment. Role models may develop into mentors, but they are usually people whose behavior is emulated. Role models and mentors are not formally fostered in nursing curricula, therefore their presence is spontaneous rather than incorporated into nursing practice as fundamental personnel.

As mentoring becomes more commonly used in health practice settings, nurses can identify role models early in their careers who demonstrate attributes to adopt. These role models can be approached, where personalities seem compatible, and the role models developed into mentors.

Mentoring is a management, nursing, and interpersonal tool to be used in professional career development. As the mentor guides the new manager in coping with multifaceted professional and managerial issues, the new manager has a teacher and counselor. The new manager who has a mentor as a model can then create an environment of excellence and self-actualization in the staff. Autonomy provided by the mentor can be translated to the staff when mentoring a new manager. This develops into nurses feeling connected and facilitates effective team building. A group of staff members who perform with excellence, supported by their manager, feel that connection in their group interactions.

As these connections build confidence needed to set higher goals, future nurses and managers welcome role models and mentors and their influence on the professional nurse manager's actualization.

SUMMARY

The new nurse manager may feel overwhelmed after the 'honeymoon' period and as the realities and constraints of daily group management are identified. Early adoption of a leadership style that is effective for both staff and manager provides order and security in a highly stressful atmosphere. Consistency and objectivity with the staff creates an environment of stability that can foster further growth and a higher level of professionalism.

Professionalism includes experienced nurses and managers mentoring new nurses and new managers. Nursing may not have promoted this concept as well as has been documented in the business world, and despite the popular notion of nurses as nurturers, nurses have not always been supportive of or encouraging about development of each other's leadership qualities. Mentoring, whether formal or informal, must be considered, as is continuing education, a professional responsibility.

REFERENCES

1. McGregor D: *Leadership and motivation,* Cambridge, 1983, MIT Press.
2. Bethel SM: *Making a difference: 12 qualities that make you a leader,* New York, 1990, GP Putnam and Sons.
3. Dunham J, Fisher E: Nurse executive profile of excellent nursing leadership, *Nurs Admin Q* 15:4, 1990.
4. Dunham J, Klafehn K: Transformational leadership and the nurse executive, *J Nurs Adm* 20:28, 1990.
5. Gillies DA: *Nursing management: a systems approach,* Philadelphia, 1989, WB Saunders.
6. Gillies DA: *Nursing management: a systems approach,* Philadelphia, 1989, WB Saunders.
7. Hersey P, Blanchard K: *Management of organizational behavior: utilizing human resources,* Englewood Cliffs, NJ, 1988, Prentice Hall.
8. Fiedler F, Chemers M: *Improving leadership effectiveness,* New York, 1984, John Wiley & Sons.
9. Tannenbaum R, Schmidt W: How to choose a leadership pattern, *Harvard Bus Rev* 51:164, 1973.
10. Stivers C: Why can't a woman be less like a man? *J Nurs Adm* 21:51, 1991.
11. Orem D: *Nursing concepts of practice,* New York, 1971, McGraw-Hill.
12. McGregor D: *The human side of enterprise,* New York, 1960, McGraw-Hill.
13. Kiely M: Nursing management brief, *Nurs Manage* 3:15, 1989.
14. Flarey DL: Redesigning management roles, *J Nurs Adm* 21:44, 1991.
15. Gillies DA: *Nursing management: a systems approach,* Philadelphia, 1989, WB Saunders.

CHAPTER **3**

Human Resource Management

T. M. Marrelli

Personnel decisions and issues can be some of the most challenging episodes of any managerial career. Conversely, the effective use of human management skills can be the highlight of your professional career. With this in mind, this chapter emphasizes the latter. It is important to note that we all improve and grow through practice. This is especially true in personnel or human resource (HR) management functions. According to Patz and others,[1] a national survey of academic health chief nurse executives and nurse managers demonstrated that human management skills were considered the most important criterion of effectiveness. Flexibility, negotiation, and compromise were second.

WHAT IS HUMAN RESOURCE MANAGEMENT?

Simply put, HR management can be defined as effective interpersonal communications between all levels of employees and staff.

TEN VITAL HR POINTS

✔ Hiring and other personnel decisions are some of the most important decisions made as a manager.

✔ You make better, more informed decisions as you gain experience.

✔ HR issues must be addressed and dealt with effectively; usually they will not be solved without interpersonal action or intervention.

✔ You cannot communicate too often; convey unit and organizational goals, constructive or positive feedback (including a thank you for a job well done), or any issue affecting the staff's work.

✔ Remember that all work is done through the staff. This is the core of HR management.

✔ Familiarize yourself with your organization's policy and procedure manuals dealing with HR issues.

✔ Remember, you are not alone. The problems surfacing on your unit have occurred before and there is a standard procedure for you to follow. Integrate the knowledge from these manuals into daily practice in your area.

✔ When making personnel decisions, particularly hiring ones, consider your unit needs (e.g., the organization, staffing patterns, care delivery system, types of patients or clients, shifts offered, benefit packages, tuition reimbursement for professional staff, and the type of nursing or administrative experience needed). Prioritize these needs.

✔ Use all resources and experts available to you for your growth as a manager in this important area. For example, if special HR department professionals or nurse recruiter professionals are available, use their services and expertise. This is especially true for areas where state or federal laws apply and you may not be aware or have the in-depth knowledge needed to interpret or implement these laws in your setting. Examples of these areas include equal opportunity employment concerns, workman compensation questions, benefit compensation issues, and other areas of a specialized nature.

This chapter is organized into the format followed in the employment process. Therefore the discussion begins with the interviewing process and proceeds to hiring, orientation, and ongoing personnel concerns.

INTERVIEWING

FIVE PREPARATION TIPS FOR A SUCCESSFUL INTERVIEW

✔ Read any facility manuals available on the process. There may be factors unique to your setting.

✔ Plan for the interview. This is vital to an effective interview for both parties. This is usually done by clearly defining your unit needs before the actual interview. This is the most important part of the interview. The applicant who cannot understand your needs may make incorrect assumptions and accept the position but leave shortly thereafter, disillusioned and angry. Example questions include: Do you need a nurse who has been or wants to be cross-trained in a particular specialty area? Do you need an experienced hospice nurse with specialized symptom management expertise? Try to define succinctly what your patient area needs to function more effectively.

✔ Plan your discussion and the specific questions and topics to be addressed.

✔ Arrange to have your phone calls held and other interruptions deferred until the interview is complete. This demonstrates to applicants that you respect them and value their time.

✔ Schedule someone to be in charge during your interview. This is particularly important if you schedule consecutive interviews.

27 TIPS ON CONDUCTING A SUCCESSFUL INTERVIEW

An effective interview allows the parties to clearly communicate and allots enough uninterrupted time that the interviewee is comfortable. Both parties should meet their common objectives of exchanging information.

✔ Start on time. Do not keep the applicant waiting because this is not a sign of power, but of rudeness. If you are not punctual, be professional and apologetic and say it was a patient emergency.

✔ Remember how you felt when you were interviewed for your last position and what was said that put you at ease.

✔ Clearly define at the beginning of the interview the time allotted for the interview. For example, "I know personnel told you this interview would be approximately 1 hour. We need to cover the important information and wrap up by 2 PM because I have a meeting immediately following our interview."

✔ Protect yourself by avoiding statements or words that may lead to accusations of sex or other types of discrimination. Common examples, very well known to most woman nurses, include *honey, sweetie,* and *dear*.

✔ Do not inquire about spouses, children (or plans for children), day-care situations, or other sensitive areas.

✔ Treat everyone the same.

✔ Be professional, kind, and a good listener. The better your active listening skills, the more information you receive from the applicant.

✔ When possible, use open-ended questions to elicit an open response. Ask about common problem situations and how the applicant would resolve them.

✔ Use silence; this allows the applicant to share more information.

✔ Remember first impressions do count, so make it a good one. You may want this applicant to want to work on your team.

✔ Be enthusiastic and talk about the good things happening on your unit or area.

✔ Give a walking tour of the clinical area and of the institution, when appropriate.

✔ Provide a brochure on your program or health setting. Use the information listed as general information to relax the applicant initially or as points of discussion during the interview.

✔ Dress professionally and neatly. If the interview is in your office, remember your office reflects you and the organization.

✔ Talk about the orientation program for new staff.

✔ Discuss the day-to-day operational aspects of the position.

✔ Elicit from the applicants why they are applying for this job. Though this sounds simple, the responses are rarely as simple.

✔ Validate the applicants' understanding of the position.

✔ Discuss the time frame in which you would like to fill the position.

✔ Ask where applicants would like to be or see themselves in 5 years.

✔ Bring applicants back for another interview when appropriate.

✔ Talk about the staff development program.

✔ Discuss the type of documentation used in your unit or area.

✔ Discuss the dress code requirements of the position.

✔ Summarize what will happen next at the conclusion. For example, "I have interviews scheduled through. . . . I hope to have the process completed by. . . ." (specify time frame or date).

✔ When appropriate, have the nurse recruiter or your staff interview your final candidate(s).

✔ For managerial candidates (e.g., assistant nurse manager), have members of your staff interview the final applicant(s).

HIRING A NEW TEAM MEMBER

Congratulations! You successfully sold yourself and your organization and you now have a new staff member. Hopefully, your staff was involved in the process and welcomes this new nurse. There are steps you can take to ensure a smooth transition for new staff members.

Making a new staff member feel welcome and part of the group is the key to long-term employee satisfaction. The ideas in the accompanying tip list are simple yet important in making your unit a place where new staff feel comfortable and grow professionally.

TIPS FOR WELCOMING A NEW STAFF MEMBER

✔ Show the new staff member his or her personal space. This can include the locker, mailbox, phone message slot, or other areas. Make sure to clearly mark his or her name, spelled correctly, on such items.

✔ Schedule the new staff member to have lunch with those members of your staff who are role models to the group.

✔ Have the new staff nurse's identification badge and access/security card completed as soon as possible.

✔ Schedule a lunch with all other new professional nursing staff. This peer camaraderie leads to job satisfaction. It also teaches the new staff members about other aspects of your facility or setting.

✔ Schedule and lead a personalized walking tour for the new nurse.

✔ Introduce the new nurse to key personnel and others encountered during the tour.

✔ Discuss the hospital-wide buddy or mentor system.

✔ Allot time in your schedule at least three times a week (even if for a few minutes) for the first few months to check on the new staff member's progress. Delegate this responsibility to a trusted nurse leader on your staff if you will be unavailable. This is also a good time to ask if what you said in the interview holds true in practice. This will help you tailor comments to future applicants.

✔ Write a welcome note to the new staff member and have other staff members sign the note.

✔ Hold a breakfast or lunch meeting so all staff members can meet the new nurse. This is particularly important in practice areas where the staff is rarely together, such as a home health agency or a community-based hospice.

✔ Personally spend time with the new staff nurse, especially introducing her to other team members in the organization at all levels.

✔ Create a phone list for new staff members. Alphabetize the list by first names. (Everyone else can remember the new nurse's first and last names, but it is unrealistic to expect the new nurse to remember all other staff members' last names immediately.)

ORIENTATION FOR NEW STAFF MEMBERS

Orientation is the time when the new staff member should become an integral part of your team. The more effort expended initially in this endeavor, the better the result, which is a more effective and autonomous nurse. Oftentimes, it feels as though the nurse is away from the unit "too long" in orientation. The more skills and knowledge that can be taught, used, and integrated into practice, the more successful this nurse will be, both to the manager and the nurse herself. Remember, you get out of people, or staff, only what you expect. Studies have shown that the manager's expectations are the key to the staff's behavior and development. Livingston,[2] who has studied this "Pygmalion" performance, states that, "The way managers treat their subordinates is subtly influenced by what they expect of them. If managers' expectations are high, productivity is likely to be excellent. If their expectations are low, productivity is likely to be poor. It is as though there were a law that caused subordinates' performance to rise or fall to meet managers' expectations."

With this information in mind, it is important to note that your enthusiasm (or apathy) are contagious, and work output is directly related to the level of managerial expectation. Use this important imformation to your advantage.

A NEW STAFF MEMBER ORIENTATION CHECKLIST

Professional nurses practice in so many settings that it is not possible to list all areas that must be covered with the new nurse. This list contains the most common themes. Some items mentioned are clearly specialized areas of practice.

✔ Benefit; compensation packages; including medical and dental policies (including when coverage begins); malpractice; licensure; professional in-service credits; physical, overtime, and compensation time policies; other benefits

✔ Leave allotments, including vacation, sick days, holidays, other leave

✔ Frequency and schedule of paydays

✔ Savings plans available (e.g., thrift or credit union)

✔ Position description

✔ Hours of shifts, specific time to report, check-in procedures, break times

✔ Uniform requirements and any associated compensation, name tag or access/security badge

✔ Employee assistance program availability

✔ Personalized orientation schedule, including clinical demonstrations, CPR, and other educational resources specific to clinical practice

✔ An in-depth personalized tour

✔ Availability and hours of organization's day care facility and/or benefits.

✔ Confidentiality policies

✔ The nursing philosophy

✔ The state's Nurse Practice Act

✔ The written standards of care

✔ Schedule of probationary and ongoing performance appraisal evaluation(s)

✔ On-call schedule and compensation process for on-call

✔ Supply acquisition and process for change

✔ The committees that the unit or staff are represented on and the process for input into change

✔ Clinical and administrative policies and procedures

✔ The facility or program mission statement and objectives

✔ Safety or risk management policies—can include security (both patient and staff) Occupational Safety and Health Administration (OSHA), Centers for Disease Control (CDC), or other safety concerns (e.g., fire or disaster plans, universal precautions, seat belt use for staff members driving in the community)

✔ Clinical documentation orientation, including forms, type and frequency of documentation required, paper flow, and an introduction to the nursing computer system

✔ Quality improvement processes

✔ Distribution and stocking of initial supplies for nurse bags in the community or other outreach setting (e.g., maps, resources available after office hours, report processes, use of pagers, car phones, and mileage reimbursement forms)

The clearer the instructions and direction provided in the orientation period, the fewer problems you will usually face in the future. Therefore the extra time you take in the beginning will pay off. You will not have to be continually clarifying rules. When you communicate rules or important information, use direct eye contact, be professional, and restate the specifics that need to be understood by both parties. There is nothing worse than a nurse saying, "I was never told that," when the subject relates to an important part of the job or could have caused a poor patient outcome. For this reason, another nurse whose judgement and skills you trust should be "a buddy" with the new nurse during the formal orientation period. In some settings this person is called a preceptor. This delegation accomplishes three things: it (1) behaviorally demonstrates your trust in your staff; (2) frees you up from day-to-day operational orientation; and (3) develops the managerial skills of the staff nurse to whom you have delegated the preceptor responsibility. This type of delegation of responsibility empowers your staff and helps them to achieve more personally and professionally.

There are two main methods of ongoing communication once the official orientation or probationary period is completed. They are (1)

counseling or coaching and (2) staff development. Both processes are equally important in different ways. These two major communication methods are discussed below.

Coaching

We would all love to work in a setting where everyone, once adequately oriented, functioned smoothly on automatic pilot. Unfortunately, this is not realistic. However, there have been occasions where nurse managers have chosen and groomed a special group of self-motivated nurses who worked together and addressed issues and reached consensuses together so effectively that it felt that way. This then can be our realistic goal.

But until we reach that point, ongoing training and reeducation must occur to reach professional and program goals. Counseling is oftentimes the vehicle for this needed communication. This is why initial (i.e., during orientation) positive communications are usually valued over corrective action, which is how counseling is frequently perceived. Unfortunately, counseling is considered negative by some managers. However, some managers perceive counseling as an opportunity to lobby, or, in effect, to identify individual problem behaviors before they become or effect staff trends. In addition, it is in the one-to-one encounters with staff members when the effective manager oftentimes learns information informally that assists in unit or program planning. With this in mind, it is important that effective counseling skills be addressed.

25 TIPS FOR EFFECTIVE COACHING OR COUNSELING

✔ Look at counseling as positive and as a challenge.

✔ Visualize yourself as being good at it.

✔ Remember, expect the best and chances are your staff will live up to your expectations.

✔ Always address an identified behavior problem sooner than later.

✔ Do not attempt to counsel or reprimand staff in front of other people.

✔ Respect the staff's right to disagree with your assessment of the situation.

✔ Be objective. When discussing an incident use the factual *who, what, when,* and *where* queries that reporters use.

✔ Try to not allow your feelings to color your input or behavior. If you are very angry or irritated, it is usually better to talk at a later time.

✔ Do not overreact. Talk to a peer manager or a mentor for input before the session and imagine and act how that calm and effective role model would in the same situation.

✔ Write up the objective behavior and the other documentation before the meeting so the plan is appropriate to the problem and you anticipate the desired outcome.

✔ Set a time limit on the discussion. For example, "Lisa, as I said at the start of our meeting we have 15 minutes, so now we need to wrap-up in 5 minutes."

✔ Use listening skills and silence to help you understand the problem and the solution.

✔ Summarize the discussion and the outcomes or plan of action clearly and succinctly.

✔ Try to schedule the session at a time and in an environment free of interruptions.

✔ Conversely, if this employee has a long-standing pattern of behavioral infractions and does not listen to time or other limits you set, control your environment by setting up planned interruptions (e.g., have someone page you.) Do not reinforce the employee's behavior by putting up with it.

✔ Treat all staff members the same; be consistent and thorough.

✔ Practice the skill of not being defensive and always try to see the other's point of view.

✔ Use the same documentation format for all staff members. Some health settings have their own counseling forms. Many use the SOAP format with very good results. (An example can be found on p. 59.)

✔ Determine what infractions at your place of employment are cause for verbal or written warnings.

✔ Be a prudent nurse and document all coaching sessions. In addition, any written anecdotal notes or documentation of critical incidents will assist in your objective feedback and recall for performance appraisals. Use this written documentation as a reminder to yourself by keeping it in the staff member's personnel folder. Remember, awards, counseling, and other discussions are written objective reminders when it is performance evaluation time.

✔ Try to follow up counseling with another scheduled session. Hopefully, the problem is resolved and you will be giving positive feedback to the employee at the second meeting.

✔ Remember that effective employee counseling does modify behavior (but the employee has to want to modify his or her behavior).

✔ Always try to end these sessions on a positive note.

✔ Believe that all employees want to do a good job.

✔ Give feedback to all staff members on a regular, frequent basis.

An Example of Coaching Documentation

The following example of unacceptable behavior is one that you may see; it would negatively affect other staff members and the smooth operation of your unit. This problem is with a new staff nurse who is 2 months out of formal orientation. She spends the first 20 minutes of many mornings trying to change the assignment you made. She does this in front of the entire change-of-shift and, it always seems, on mornings when you have a crisis that occurred during the evening shift and that needs to be documented by you and placed on your supervisor's desk immediately. This behavior gets all of your unit off to a bad start (and it's not even 7:30 AM). In her favor, you are well aware of this nurse's capabilities and, though she is relatively new, you know she is very strong clinically and already acts as an informal leader to the group.

You are an effective manager in that you (1) identify a problem behavior, (2) address it early and when you are not angry, and (3) ask her privately to stop by your office in 10 minutes (this is effective so the staff member does not worry more and come in defensive and upset). It is 7:40 AM and she comes into your office. Following is an example of the documentation that addresses what occurred in the meeting and the joint plan for resolution.

S(ubjective): Ms. Davis says, "I don't know why I do that every morning. I don't like my assignment. I still think though that Mrs. Smith should stay with Nurse Carter and I should get Mr. Jones since he has cancer and you know I'm in school to become a clinical specialist in oncology."

O(bjective): 7:40 AM, 12/15/93, Ms. Davis is in my office after two previous informal *(list dates, when known)* discussions with her about the same topic: wanting to revamp the patient assignments totally. Today specifically there were two nurses upset because they told me they were still not sure what their assignments were—and this was after report. Ms. Davis was calm and clearly stated that she transferred 2 months ago to care primarily for cancer patients.

A(ssessment): Situation leaves the staff feeling unsettled and compromises patient care by the nonproductive time spent haggling over assignments. After an open discussion with Ms. Davis, she believes I am not respecting her area of expertise and that she had the understanding when she transferred to this unit that she would care primarily for oncologic and hospice patients.

P(lan): Ms. Davis verbally validated that she understands how this behavior is not conducive to a team effort in caring for patients and why some of the nurses have discussed the problem with me. The plan we agreed on is as follows: when possible, I will assign her cancer patients. However, she verbalizes understanding of changing staffing needs and will accept assignments without comment or further discussion starting tomorrow at morning report. In addition, she asked that I investigate the possibility of her being cross-trained to the organization's affiliated hospice program. She stated that she believes this would allow more flexibility and perhaps continuity of care for some of our unit's in-patients. We will meet next Tuesday at this time to follow up on our plan and to validate that the complaining sessions have stopped as demonstrated by timely acceptance of assignments delegated.

The documentation of employee performance demonstrated specific, objective behaviors that necessitated the meeting. As shown in this example, training needs are often identified through effective counseling. In these sessions, both parties should feel better; the manager, who will see a positive behavior change because of the information learned in the session, and the employee, who sees that the effective manager identified training needs that will help the organization and the nurse's professional goals. These training needs are best met in ongoing staff development programs.

Staff Development

An effective staff development program and expert clinicians are vital to nursing growth, satisfaction, and a quality care environment. Orientation, planned in-house services, and continuing education programs all support an effective staff development program. With the constant development of myriad clinical breakthroughs, new technology, legislation, and other factors, professional nurses must be kept up to date. These educational encounters help ensure nursing maintains recognized standards of practice. In addition, a well planned and executed staff development program is valued highly by staff. The effective new nurse manager recognizes that allowing staff specialization through continuing education is an adjunct to her role modeling and facilitates staff attendance, thus behaviorally reinforcing the value of ongoing education and training in professional practice.

FIRING OR LETTING GO OF A STAFF MEMBER

Probably no management decision is as difficult to be involved in as the process of firing an employee. In most institutions, firing is the last resort. In rare instances, this process has been in the works for some time, but the infractions needing to be documented or personnel's policies were not effective until the new nurse manager arrived. Should such a serious and ongoing problem be yours, share this responsibility with both your immediate supervisor and the personnel manager. There are legal concerns, staff ramifications, confidentiality issues, and other areas that should be addressed by others with the needed expertise in your system. In most settings, these situations occur only with the concurrence and involvement of the HR manager. In all cases, it is a difficult process for all involved. Because of this, you should not handle this process without adequate support and direction, particularly in a situation that has been ongoing for some time and began before your tenure.

EVALUATING PERFORMANCE

Generally, no area creates more feelings between manager and staff members than the performance evaluation or appraisal process. Because it is often tied to money and self-esteem, it may become the focus of some disagreement between supervisor and employee. An effective performance evaluation is beneficial to both the manager and the staff member being evaluated. In addition, the performance evaluation should be a written validation of what the manager and employee have been discussing and documenting throughout the period before the formal process. Sadly, this is not always the case and so the employee feels and has a right to complain that the manager did not communicate problems to the employee before the meeting.

Usually there is a formal structure for the process and a timeframe for appraising performance. Most facilities or settings also have a standard format and criteria on which to base the evaluation. It is very important that you learn the organization's evaluation process. Various evaluation tools are available, and you need to familiarize yourself with them. The purpose of this section is to prepare you for your first employee performance evaluation or to reinforce information if you have previously administered evaluations.

What is Performance Appraisal?

Performance appraisals occur to (1) give formal feedback on the current nursing performance in the work setting and (2) determine the employee's development within the staff or other growth needs for the future. This is provided in a private discussion and can be a positive experience for both nurse manager and employee.

Though the process and time-frames may vary, common elements among successful and effective performance appraisals exist and are as follows:

- They provide needed recognition and structured feedback.
- They allow the manager and staff nurse time to reevaluate the bigger picture of organization, unit direction, or goals.
- They allow the nurse manager to clarify behavior or other expectations.

- They allow the staff nurse a reading on her defined or written priorities, goals, and objectives.
- Evaluations permit the nurse manager another opportunity to create an environment that fosters personal and professional growth of staff nurses in an open environment that encourages risk taking, where appropriate.
- The process is another time when the nurse manager can allow the exchange of creative ideas to accomplish work in a different or better way.
- It can be an opportunity to coach the nurse employee to meet program or unit goals or objectives.
- Sometimes, evaluations are the environment for addressing the core of why we choose to be nurses. For example, discussions of effectiveness, professionalism, client relations, clinical expertise, and other factors all determine the level of the performance appraisal. All nurses and employees want to do a good job—this is a unique opportunity to find out what is impeding the employee's attainment of goals and what you can do as the manager to facilitate goal achievement. This role as coach and mentor solidifies your working relationship with your staff.
- Evaluations allow the quality of the work performance to be evaluated against specific predetermined standards that are correlated with the employee position description.

SUMMARY

The manager must effectively employ human management skills to achieve work objectives. The use of these skills, or their lack, is evident in any work environment. As the role model for the staff, it is imperative that the new nurse manager have an open attitude that creates a workplace where staff nurses can grow professionally. An effective workplace has the following qualities:

1. It is an environment open to new ideas.
2. Staff members feel they can safely take risks, when appropriate.
3. Planning occurs for short- and long-term activities and the staff is involved and apprised.
4. Both management and the staff are working toward the same goals.
5. All levels of staff value human management skills and treat everyone, including peers, patients, and visitors, with kindness and respect.

As a nurse manager, these are the elements to strive for in your setting. The important HR functions of interviewing, hiring, coaching, and evaluating performance are the hallmarks of the team's inception and structure.

Please see Chapter 4, Communications, for a discussion of specific communication problems that may arise in HR management.

REFERENCES

1. Patz JM, Biordi DL, Holm K: Middle Nurse Manager Effectiveness, *J Nurs Admin* 21:15, 1991.

2. Livingson J, Sterling, HBR: Pygmalion in Management, *Harvard Bus Rev* 66:121, 1988.

CHAPTER 4

Communications

Margaret Sharp Woodard
T. M. Marrelli

RECOGNIZING YOUR INHERENT INTERPERSONAL SKILLS

Managers can perform multitudes of tasks proficiently, effectively select and hire staff, delegate appropriately, make sound decisions, and yet still not achieve maximal success. Strong, well developed interpersonal skills are a key to all management functions. Interpersonal skills are a large element of the art and science of effective management. These skills are necessary in the development of trust and mutual respect between manager and staff members. This trust and respect foster staff development and retention and can minimize the effect of negative events such as times of high stress or change.

Interpersonal skills can be learned. Yet we all have "inherent" interpersonal abilities that affect our success as managers. Elements of personality and style are unique to each individual. Successful use of interpersonal skills is varied and adapted to the specific situation. Reading, noting instances of effective communication, and seeking feedback from supervisors and the staff are all methods nurse managers can use to analyze the impact and effectiveness of their "inherent" qualities. Through thoughtful self-examination, it is possible to temper or emphasize personal characteristics to enhance your success and meet management goals. Some nurse managers naturally exhibit warmth and inspire liking and trust. Some have an innate ability to excite and inspire the staff and others to do well. Although these gifts assist managers, the gifts must be accompanied by learned interpersonal skills and sound managerial skills and abilities. We all have probably known ineffective managers with great charm.

Conversely, many of us do not have a personality or style that gives us rapid acceptance or strong impact. It is important to remember that long-term effectiveness need not be diminished in this situation. Fairness, good judgement, accomplishment, and communication will eventually establish a true foundation of the trust and respect needed by all nurse managers to succeed.

The analysis of your skills and abilities allows you to use them to your advantage, develop complementary skills, and compensate for weaker areas. An example of this was an experienced nurse manager with great organizational and systems skills who appeared cold and directive. In previous jobs, she had discovered that this tended to shut her off from the staff. It took her many years to win their trust, and she often experienced knee-jerk resistance to and suspicion of new ideas or recommendations. Over time, this decreased as staff began to recognize the benefits and results of her abilities. In her next job she compensated for such a reception early on by telling the staff that she realized she was often perceived as difficult to approach and lacking in warmth. She asked them to look past this initial impression and give her time to demonstrate caring and open-mindedness through her actions and work. She worked hard to consistently reward those who approached her. She also hired an assistant head nurse with a warmer, more open attitude. These actions worked toward decreasing the negative impact her natural manner tended to create.

While recognizing the importance of building rapport, trust, and a support base, the nurse manager must realize that her goal is not to be universally liked or popular.

There are learnable techniques of communication, leadership, development, and motivation of staff that are components of interpersonal skills. These are discussed in the remainder of the chapter.

HOW TO GET WHAT YOU WANT

Interpersonal skills help you get what you want to achieve organizational work. This occurs directly, through clear communication, and indirectly, by creating an environment for open, trusting communication.

Know What You Want: Goals and Values

To get what you want, you and your staff must know specifically what you want. The first step is to establish clear, mutually accepted values. In most nursing settings, the focus of these values is directed toward providing quality patient care. It can be extremely useful to discuss and clarify with staff members what is valued and how those values are supported and demonstrated. Once consensus and clarity concerning values are reached, they should be frequently reviewed. Most nurses are stimulated by and interested in this type of discussion. It causes them to remember why they became nurses and to examine their practice, work habits, and routines in a new light.

After values are clearly defined, future decisions and discussions of goals, standards, and performance should be guided by these values. Clearly stated goals for patient care, unit function, and individual staff members must be established. The goals should be valued, measurable, and achievable. They should be developed using institutional, departmental, and regulatory guidelines, policies, and objectives. Staff members should always have input. Although goals should be achievable and realistic, they should also be challenging. Much productivity and pride in achievement is lost when goals are set at a low level. Relating unit goals to values concerning patient care is important. It is easier to set and strive for high-level goals when the effect on patients, if goals are not achieved, is clear and demonstrable.

The Nurse Manager Role

As the manager, your role in defining values and setting goals includes the following:

- Initiating and facilitating discussion to elicit clarification of values.
- Recording written value statements, seeking staff feedback, and incorporating revision.
- Initiating discussion of goals at the unit and individual levels with the staff you directly supervise.
- Bringing pertinent directives, regulations, or other factors needing consideration to the discussion.
- Recording written goals and action plans for achieving them.
- Maintaining momentum of progress toward goals, giving positive and constructive feedback to promote progress toward meeting deadlines.

DEVELOPING RESOURCES

Clear goals and values assist the nurse manager and nursing staff in finding direction and setting priorities. To reach these goals, the nurse manager must develop, maintain, conserve, and wisely use both personnel and material resources. The development and retention of employees involves important interpersonal skills in any setting and time. They are crucial in the nursing profession. Advanced, more complex practice requires experienced nurses. The demands for efficiency can only be met with a complement of staff members who are familiar with unit and ancillary systems. Nurses today are in high demand, and the turnover created as they seek new opportunities is expensive in dollars, productivity, and training.

Each staff member on any unit is a resource to be highly valued. The nurse manager must have individual knowledge of every employee directly supervised and ongoing communication with those indirectly supervised. There are several purposes of this communication and knowledge.

The first purpose is to identify the skill level and learning needs of the staff. Psychomotor skills, critical clinical thinking, and the ability to plan and deliver care should be assessed. Knowledge of individual learning styles should be incorporated into planning for the development of each individual. Professional staff members should be involved in developing their own plan and take responsibility for their learning.

THE IMPORTANCE OF JOB SATISFACTION

Another key reason for the nurse manager to develop relationships with and knowledge of each staff member is that this increases the ability to maximize staff job satisfaction. While the nurse manager must balance unit function against individual needs, there are many opportunities to assist staff in enjoying their work. Most nurses today balance family and individual demands against those of their career. A person who enjoys her work and workplace can be energized rather than drained by her work (on most days!). This allows the career person to carry energy rather than fatigue out of the workplace. It also leads her to value that particular job setting enough to be less likely to leave it for other than serious career reasons.

Mark Twain is reported to have defined the successful person as one who gets up in the morning and is excited to meet each day. When a job contributes to that feeling, one is not likely to move on. Many nurses today indicate that they leave their jobs because of boredom, poor work conditions, lack of opportunity, inability to advance, interpersonal conflicts, and conflict with personal needs.

THE NURSE MANAGER'S ROLE IN STAFF RETENTION

The nurse manager must understand the factors that satisfy or dissatisfy staff members to retain staff. Five examples of using this knowledge to retain your staff and create a healthier workplace follow.

Example One

An assistant head nurse approached the nurse manager about a trio of staff members. She was concerned because they tended to work together and adjust their assignments and schedules to accommodate this goal. She was worried that this might adversely affect productivity. The three were skilled, competent, and experienced nurses. One historically had a problem with absenteeism and another was previously a loner. On further discussion with the manager, it became clear that these nurses were completing assignments, were not disruptive to others, were not cliquish, and were enjoying working together. They functioned as an effective, cooperative team. Their patients had good outcomes. The assistant head nurse was worried because of vague feelings that sociability at work should be limited and sensed some loss of control. She was encouraged by the manager to examine this situation for actual, objective, negative results and could identify none. They then explored possible positive effects such as increased collaboration, support, and affiliation. After further discussion, the assistant head nurse approached the three and remarked on their pattern. She verbalized appreciation of practice and collaboration, and support for its benefits. She encouraged them to continue, but discussed concerns about productivity. All agreed that patient care was the priority. Over time several benefits were seen: (1) the nurse with an absenteeism problem rarely called in sick because she did not want to let her friends down; (2) the three became very involved in unit orientation, and their skills and warmth were excellent for new staff members; and (3) the group also became a nucleus for unit social activities, as well as special projects—they worked so well together that they had very good ideas to share with others.

SKILLS USED BY THE NURSE MANAGER

- Recognized staff and what motivates them
- Reinforced positive behaviors
- Verbalized appreciation of practice and collaboration

Example Two

A nurse manager met with an excellent RN who had been with the unit for 2 years. The nurse was clinically skilled but not very involved in unit issues outside of completing her work in a given shift. Historically, 2 years was the average turnover time for this particular unit. The manager and nurse explored the nurse's goals. The nurse liked the patient care setting but was in need of new stimulation and growth. They both agreed that she was not ready for a management position, nor was one available. After discussion, the nurse accepted an assignment to develop and implement patient teaching protocols for her area of clinical expertise. The manager met with her regularly to review progress, offer support, and assist her in obtaining needed resources. The nurse was later selected for a hospital-wide committee, which furthered her growth and development. She became very active on the unit by sharing her new skills and acting as a resource to peers.

SKILLS USED BY THE NURSE MANAGER

- Identified staff member's goals
- Listened and created an environment that allowed the nurse to grow professionally
- Scheduled regular meetings to review progress, offer support, and assist in obtaining resources

---

Example Three

The nurse manager met with a staff member who was going to school to advance from LPN to RN. She worked full-time. They discussed ways to accommodate her class schedule without disrupting the unit or staff schedule. She was given time frames for discussing scheduling needs in advance. At one point, it became clear that she would be 30 minutes late 2 days a week on the evening shift. She and the manager discussed options. As report was one-to-one on this unit, she was encouraged to approach others who might swap an hour during the week to be relieved 1 hour early on the weekend. This plan was successful for the nurse, the nurse manager, and the entire unit.

SKILLS USED BY THE NURSE MANAGER

- Behaviorally supported a staff member's professional growth
- Listened and implemented a plan based on staff member's goal
- Discussed option for scheduling

Example Four

The charge nurse on a step-down unit approached her nurse manager to discuss advancing her own critical care skills. The manager arranged for her to have access to an ICU preceptor. The charge nurse scheduled herself to spend time in the ICU when her shift was covered. She and the manager regularly discussed her progress and use of time. At the end of 6 months, the charge nurse in-serviced other staff on new procedures and began scheduling them for similar off-unit development.

SKILLS USED BY THE NURSE MANAGER

- Supported professional autonomy by having the nurse schedule herself
- Arranged access for the staff member to the ICU preceptor
- Discussed regularly progress and time use

Example Five

While meeting with a staff member, a manager discovered that an important part of her life was attending a Tuesday evening meeting. Without inconveniencing other staff, but with some effort on adjusting the schedule, the manager thereafter scheduled this nurse off on that evening whenever possible. The manager later discovered that of many more difficult tasks she performed on behalf of her staff, this was one of the most appreciated.

SKILLS USED BY THE NURSE MANAGER

- Listened to and heard the staff nurse's need
- Altered the schedule to support the nurse's request
- Respected the staff member by implementing this change

In the above examples the managers were successful in developing and retaining staff. The key to these simple but successful examples is that the managers' responses were individualized to the specific circumstances and individuals. Some management situations do not lend themselves to a single strategy and require ongoing evaluation and support for successful resolution. Most important, development and retention of staff can occur consistently only in an environment where each individual is valued and appreciated. This is demonstrated through action and verbalization by the effective nurse manager.

USING RESOURCES: MOTIVATION

We know that clarifying values, setting clear goals, and developing resources are important in a successful operation. Nurse managers must also use resources effectively. In the case of personnel resources, this requires motivation coupled with effective leadership. Remember, all work is done by the staff.

Lancaster[1] defines motivation as internal and unique to each employee. In other words, managers cannot motivate employees, they must be motivated from within, and what inspires motivation in one may not in another. Lancaster states that all employees are motivated, but those who appear to lack motivation are actually motivated in a direction different, or toward other outcomes, than a manager may desire. Because managers cannot directly motivate staff, they must work indirectly by creating an environment that tends to cause individual motivation toward the desired goals.

TIPS TO HELP CREATE A MOTIVATING ENVIRONMENT

We have discussed several activities that are part of a motivating environment. The following tips will help the nurse manager create a positive environment:

✔ Involve your staff through their participation and agreement on values and goals established.

✔ Get to know each staff member well enough to learn what assistance they need to achieve a goal and what constitutes a positive reward for them.

✔ Clarify, discuss, and reinforce the goals and what is expected with staff.

THE WORK ENVIRONMENT

A healthy work environment, put simply, is one where all employees, managers and staff members alike, work toward common goals, receive feedback and communications on an ongoing basis, and meet the needs of their customers.

The presence or absence of some of the characteristics described above in an environment does not, in itself, determine a "good" or "bad" setting. Some organizations may exhibit a blend of both in some situations, depending on times and areas observed. However, in a recent study of nurses and the culture of excellence in their hospitals, as defined by the attributes of excellence, identified by Peters and Waterman in an article by Kramer and Schmalenberg,[2] it was determined that "the presence of these attributes of excellence correlated with high job satisfaction and high self-esteem among the nurses."[2] In addition, when the authors looked at the data on the attributes of excellence, they saw "many more magnet hospital nurses indicated that their nursing leaders have power; that they're visionary; that they communicate and implement ideas, values, and goals; and that they function as a team."[3]

ABOUT FEEDBACK

The nurse manager should provide ongoing feedback and reinforcement concerning performance and achievement. Although feed-

---

ENVIRONMENT CHARACTERISTICS

CHARACTERISTICS OF A HEALTHY AND MOTIVATING ENVIRONMENT

Some work environments are healthy and others are not so healthy. The following list outlines common elements of healthy work environments.
- People feel part of a team.
- There is ongoing clear communication up and down the organization hierarchy.
- Everyone is aware of and works toward defined goals.
- Good behavior is valued and reinforced.
- Staff development is ongoing.
- Employees have the authority to complete their work.
- The work and the people are respected.
- The staff feels generally positive about the work and other staff.

CHARACTERISTICS OF AN UNHEALTHY ENVIRONMENT

Similarly, unhealthy work environments share some common characteristics. They are listed below.
- Divisiveness is apparent among the staff, as in a dysfunctional family ("we versus they").
- People complain continually or do not communicate at all.
- People do not want to come to work.
- New members may feel isolated.
- "Top down" communication is rare or nonexistent.
- An open-door policy is espoused but in reality is rarely practiced.
- There are continually identified problems without attempts at resolution.
- Paralysis through continual analysis is apparent, and no or very little effective action is taken.

---

back and reinforcement can be both positive and negative, Lancaster[1] suggests avoiding using threats and punishment as the predominating mode. Positive rewards and depersonalized, anticipated disciplinary action are more effective. Positive rewards should be individualized and can include raises, recognition, opportunities to participate in special activities, educational experiences, committee selection, and scheduling choices. Disciplinary action should be expected (i.e., a specific reaction to a specific behavior, consistent, timely, and focused on the behavior, not the person). It is important to remember that even discipline can occur in an atmosphere of approval and support.

COMMUNICATION PATTERNS

In any organization, both motivation and effectiveness are driven by the quality achieved in and patterns of communication. Without sound communication skills, the manager can be isolated and uninformed. Managers need to send and receive clear, well understood messages. Communication patterns that affect their ability to do this are discussed below.

The Communication Climate

In his book, Swansburg[3] discusses the importance of the overall tone of the environment in supporting clear communication, effective teamwork, and productivity. The supportive versus the defensive climate is discussed. The supportive climate is the goal of the manager who wants to encourage involvement and participation of staff at all levels. The manager must be open to disagreement, discussion, and input and use them constructively. Employees must feel they will be rewarded for speaking up, asking questions, and identifying problems. Individuality and spontaneity must be valued. Conflict should be seen as an opportunity for growth and learning. Empathy and support for and among staff should be evident. The only qualifier to these activities is that all should use them constructively to work towards unit goals.

TEN BASIC TIPS FOR COMMUNICATING EFFECTIVELY

✔ Sharpen and use your listening skills to hear also the tone and intent of what is being communicated.

✔ Use appropriate eye contact during your conversations with staff.

✔ Validate what you thought you understood or heard by repeating the message in your own words, when necessary.

✔ If you find yourself in a situation where you know you are too busy to listen and address an issue, schedule time with the staff member to focus on the concern.

✔ Create an environment where the only dumb questions are the ones that do not get asked.

✔ Encourage feedback, recommendations, and "ways to make things better."

✔ Smile when speaking with staff members whenever possible and appropriate.

✔ Summarize the conversation or discussion when finished.

✔ Ask for and thank staff and other team members for their ideas, input, and time.

✔ Be courteous and respectful of staff ideas and recommendations, even when they do not work out once implemented.

IMPEDIMENTS TO EFFECTIVE COMMUNICATIONS

Because of interference and noise, messages sent are frequently distorted before reception. Miscommunications can be caused by the sender, the listener, intermediaries, or the environment. The sender may clearly understand the message because of having had previous discussions and thoughts about the topic. The message may be poorly understood by the listener, who does not have the sender's frame of reference. The listener may produce interference simply by thinking about her response or another issue instead of listening carefully. A common example of intermediary interference is the parlor game where a phrase is whispered from person to person and the first and final messages are compared. In the game, the disparity between the first and final messages can be very amusing, but in a work setting it is a serious problem. The nurse manager must consider possible sources of communications interference in advance and eliminate as many as possible.

FOUR EXAMPLES OF WAYS TO AVOID MISCOMMUNICATIONS

✔ Communicate directly to groups.

✔ Hold meetings in a quiet setting.

✔ Encourage discussion of information given.

✔ Include a feedback loop in communication channels. After one-to-one, group, or written messages, the manager needs to ensure the message was understood as intended.

VERBAL VERSUS NONVERBAL COMMUNICATION

How something is said can be as important as what is said. Tone of voice, gestures, and posture greatly affect the listener. The nurse manager needs to appear assured, modify her feelings before speaking (or acknowledge rather than deny them), and maintain an open, attentive posture. The manager must also note body language in staff members that appears to be blocking communication. If an employee is turning away, or making a dismissive gesture, the manager must investigate or intervene at the appropriate time.

The nurse manager must always be aware of being a role model to the staff. The manager's example and behaviors must be consistent and professional. Communications should follow the formal chain of command. Nurse managers should be clear about the organization's expectations for intradepartmental and interdepartmental communications. They should make staff aware of these and their own expectations.

Inappropriate and negative forms of communication that the nurse manager should discourage in staff members and must never personally demonstrate include:

- Profanity, crudity, and personal criticisms. Professionals should express themselves professionally and demonstrate respect for others.
- Rumors and rumor spreading. Rumors can be destructive, divisive, and counterproductive.

The nurse manager serves as the vital link between the staff and the organization at large. The manager must accurately receive and transmit messages in both directions. Staff concerns, patient care issues, and system needs must be taken to administration or ancillary services. Imperatives, directives, objectives, procedures, and policies must be brought to staff. The manager uses writing, verbal, and listening skills to fulfill these linking functions. The nurse manager should review the institution's organizational chart with both supervisor and staff. The organizational chart delineates the chain of command and communication. It assists in clarifying direct, indirect, and collaborative relationships. Analysis of the chart can assist the nurse manager in ensuring that appropriate sources of information are fully used and that written and verbal communications are properly directed.

LISTENING SKILLS

It is important to remember that listening is an active process. It involves focusing, questioning, and validating, as well as allowing time to process the information gained. The listener who is judging the message or messenger, distracted, preparing a response, or not attentive cannot be listening effectively or gaining what is possible. Through meetings, nurse managers and their staffs maintain and work toward improving the function of their units. The new nurse manager needs to understand what information is important and must be noted and the process for recording such information. She needs to know how to obtain follow-up details and clarification, when needed. This clear, correct, timely information will then be communicated to all staff members. For an in-depth discussion of staff meetings, please refer to Chapter Five, "Day-to-Day Operations."

VERBAL SKILLS

Nurse managers must always be prepared to represent or speak on behalf of their clinical areas. Although one does not want to be perceived as a squeaky wheel in an era of constrained resources, the unprepared and nonverbal lose out. The successful manager can clearly articulate problems and quantify them, as well as suggest solutions. The manager should consult with supervisors, resource persons, and peers to develop the ability to speak in the language style understood and appreciated by administrators. The economic and patient outcome issues of a problem should be clearly defined. Knowing when to speak and being able to defer an answer are other important considerations. The manager does not want to be recognized for noise but for valued input. The following listed points are concepts to consider.

GUIDELINES TO CONSIDER WHEN REPRESENTING YOURSELF OR YOUR CLINICAL AREA

✔ If you do not have a complete answer for superiors or staff, say so, and commit to follow-up.

✔ Know your listener. Some people prefer a time-saving, "bottom-line" response backed up by written reinforcement or discussion. Others need a progression of thought and time.

✔ Say less. If you are clear and concise, you need not say more except to be certain you were understood. Do not dilute the message by wandering or defending. Stay on the topic if a discussion ensues.

✔ If you are not sure that you have been understood, ask your listener for feedback.

✔ Be positive and constructive. Problems can be presented in terms of needs, goals, and possible solutions. Disagreement can be presented as an alternative view while acknowledging others and encouraging comparison.

WRITTEN COMMUNICATION

The nurse manager cannot rely solely on verbal communication. Written communication provides important verification of verbal communication and discussion; access to those unavailable for meetings; documentation of standards, policies, issues, and goals; and time saving transmittal of detail and facts.

When communicating with administration and ancillary services, the manager should write a short, concise memo clearly stating the issue at hand. A memo is not the place to slowly build a case; there is too much risk of losing the reader's attention. Back-up data and explanations can be attached and referenced. The manager's supervisor should receive a copy of important memos and should be consulted about forwarding it to others.

Memo Example

In the example in the accompanying box, a specialty care unit was hampered by delayed transportation of patients. This had been discussed in many meetings, and both the manager's supervisor and the Director of Transportation were aware of the issues. The Transportation Supervisor had assured the nurse manager that problems were now corrected and insisted service was adequate. The manager and her supervisor agreed that the Director of Transport should re-

---

MEMORANDUM

DATE: November 13, 199●

TO: Alice Johnson
Transportation Supervisor

FROM: Jean Brown, Nurse Manager
Cardiac Catheterization Laboratory

RE: Transportation of patients for cardiac catheterization

Since our last meeting on October 12, I have carefully monitored transportation data to assess its effect on our patient care services. During the past month, 30 of 50 patients were delivered to the unit more than 30 minutes late, and 22 were held on the unit for longer than 45 minutes awaiting transportation after the procedure was completed.

This caused six cancellations of procedures because of lost time slots and a significant amount of overtime paid to staff to stay beyond scheduled shifts.

Patient safety was maintained, but they were quite frustrated by long waits and especially by cancellations.

Although I appreciate your efforts to improve services and also the constraints on your department, I feel we must further consider alternatives if we are to meet our goals of quality patient care. Please contact me in the next week to arrange a meeting.

Thank you.
jbw
cc: Jane Sessoms, Assistant Director
Bill Elam, Director of Transportation

---

ceive a copy of the memo but that the Transportation Supervisor should review it with the Director of Nursing.

For an in-depth discussion of memos in daily practice, please refer to Chapter 5, Day-to-Day Operations.

Other Written Products

Staff meeting minutes, recording of unit and individual goals, and performance evaluations and feedback also require written skills. Goals and evaluations are usually recorded in an institution-wide format. The manager should work with her supervisor and employees to ensure goals and evaluations are measurable, accurate, constructive, and clear. Ongoing meetings with the staff to discuss goals and progress should occur. Documentation of these meetings should reflect achievement, need for growth, and plans (in specific terms) to meet goals. This documentation will then support and verify the formal evaluation.

Staff meeting minutes are recorded to (1) ensure verbal information was heard, (2) document that all staff members received consistent information, and (3) supply detail that need not be discussed. In addition to recording attendance, minutes should be placed in a communication book or other device and signed by the staff. This is particularly important for members who were not present at the meeting. Memos, new policies and procedures, and written announcements introduced in meetings should be refered to in the minutes and placed in the book for sign-off. The manager should ensure this feedback loop is completed by all staff members by periodically reviewing for completion and giving feedback and direction as needed.

PROBLEM COMMUNICATIONS

The new nurse manager must bring or develop a wide range of skills needed for her new role. As any staff nurse or nurse manager knows, conflicts with physicians, other team members, or difficult patients and families can present their own unique problems and resolutions. Historically, nurses have been subordinate to physicians. In addition, because nursing is a predominantly female profession and medicine is a predominately male profession, gender differences can contribute to physician-nurse problems. As the numbers of female physicians and male nurses increase, physician-nurse relationships may improve. But traditional male physician domination still sometimes sets the stage for power and control games between physicians and nurses. Because of these factors, you may need your supervisor's support in the management of these conflicts. Some facilities are openly addressing these concerns by establishing nurse-physician committees. The JCAHO standard for multidisciplinary care can be the catalyst for needed changes in the relationships between health care professionals that would affect patient care positively and support increased nursing professionalism.

Communication problems are often heightened by the need for some reporting mechanism when a patient is placed at risk; for example, when a procedure is done incorrectly. A staff nurse describes the situation, "The hospital administration wants us to tell them anytime a physician contaminates a subclavian catheter during insertion. The physician knows when he's done a procedure incorrectly, and it's not my responsibility to monitor him." In this example the nurse is incorrect in her assertion. The law, including today's courts' interpretation of it, requires the nurse to pursue affirmative actions for patients and to safeguard them against incompetent health care providers. Such affirmative action—according to the courts—would, as a minimum, include monitoring the physician, even to the extent of confrontation. Otherwise, the nurse would be considered negligent."[4]

These examples and others like them bring home this ongoing problem. Like any other area in conflict resolution, the individuals involved in such a problem can usually identify and work out the most effective solutions. This is where your tact and communication skills can be put to the test. However, in those instances where the patient is jeopardized, there is only one solution. A nurse's primary duty is to the welfare of the patient, and the physician must be reported. Of course, the nurse must go through the appropriate channels in the chain of command to ensure protection of self and the patient. This is the level where the nurse manager most often becomes involved. Beyond you, the usual route is your nursing supervisor through to an administrative representative. Many times the nurse manager will clarify the situation with the physician directly. By asking the physician to explain and by getting input from others and following facility policies, particularly on the completion of incident reports, the nurse manager can follow up on known episodes where the patient was at risk.

It is important to note that some studies have demonstrated that positive professional relationships are reflected in lower patient mortality rates. Those who have been in nursing for some years know intuitively that this would be true. This concept is further explored later in this chapter.

There are positive, proactive steps the effective nurse manager can take to facilitate and maintain ongoing open communications between staff nurses and physicians. In addition, the collaboration between nurses and physicians is increasing. According to the National Joint Practice Commission,[5] "Collaborative or joint practice in hospitals is nurses and physicians collaborating as colleagues to provide patient care." Some of the ways to increase cooperation are listed below.

TECHNIQUES FOR IMPROVING NURSE-PHYSICIAN COOPERATION

✔ Establish a collaborative practice model.

✔ Provide assertiveness training for your staff, with an emphasis on clear communication skills.

✔ Be supportive by being an active listener for the nurses.

✔ Put the nursing philosophy and mission statement of your unit on the physicians' bulletin board. This can help ensure that all are working toward the same goals.

✔ Develop and implement a buddy system to achieve these goals. Assign one nurse to one new resident or physician staff member. This will help increase the new physician's comfort level and ensure a complete orientation to your unit and to "how things are done." Most new physicians will welcome the opportunity for education rather than having to face learning by trial and error. In addition, such activities assist in the achievement of mutual respect and effective communications.

✔ Hear and understand both the physicians' and nurses' positions and roles.

✔ Develop and implement an integrated documentation system (if not currently available).

✔ Establish a physician-nurse committee for (1) collaboration (patient care review); (2) problem resolution, where indicated; and (3) education regarding the role of the professional nurse in your setting.

✔ Provide ongoing education for nurses to ensure clinical expertise in care of patients. This promotes the nurse's self-esteem and is vital to effective communications or discussions with physicians about patient care.

✔ Schedule and maintain ongoing joint clinical care rounds for nurses and physicians. These are particularly important for planning care after discharge from your setting or program, considering increases in patient acuity, decreased lengths of stay, and increased patient turnover.

✔ Develop a communication process to keep physicians apprised of events, systems, or changes that affect patient care or their routines in your environment. For example, when you read your staff meeting minutes, look for these types of items. Then communicate them to the physician staff. Post a physician's board on the unit. Information to post could include (1) new products selected and available for use; (2) staff changes and promotions; (3) QA/QI issues that affect your unit; (4) any research occurring; and (5) anything else that would give information to the physician that would facilitate being a part of the team.

✔ Distribute communications about or from your area to physicians. It will help you and your staff by informing the physicians you work with in the facility. For example, some hospital-based home health agencies or hospices distribute a packet of information to new physicians on staff or physicians new to the agency. This can include a welcome letter, signed jointly by the nursing and medical directors; the philosophy; the patient admission criteria; the types of patients that would be appropriate; an example of the referral form; and a brochure on the program. Follow-up could also be arranged to personalize this interaction or to address any questions that may have been raised by the information sent.

✔ Provide ongoing physician-and-nurse educational sessions. For example, the hospice medical director, the pharmacist, and the hospice/home care nurse could provide a seminar on "effective pain relief." These clinical conferences are useful to both nurses and physicians and, as such, are important to patient care collaboration. Some other areas could be ethical dilemmas, available resources for discharge planning, and clinical updates. Be sure to evaluate these sessions to ensure that nurse and physician needs are being met. In addition, ask physicians what topic they would like addressed in the future.

✔ Post the next scheduled session and specific information on the bulletin board. Some hospitals host Grand Rounds and have well-known clinicians speak on a particular topic. They invite all physicians, nurse managers, and staff members and may have an evening meeting over dinner.

✔ Be a role model to your staff in your communications and interactions with physicians. This is particularly helpful with "difficult" physicians.

✔ Host get-togethers on a regular basis for new residents or staff physicians and nurses to begin this pattern of effective communication and role definition from the onset.

There is no question that increased collaboration of physicians and nurses will become standard in all health settings. This era of doing more with less resources ensures that we all must work together to meet patient needs. Respect must be valued and mutual for communications to be effective among all team members. We know that increased morale and "making a difference" are important in nurse satisfaction and retention. The effective nurse manager can be successful as the catalyst to create this environment.

THE WORK CULTURE

All work settings have a culture, which is the unique environment of the workplace. This culture includes the physical setting and layout, the management philosophy, and the written and unwritten rules for conduct and other activities. In nursing, the work of managing in this culture occurs in ongoing communications, usually with small groups, teams, or individual employees. A team is a group of people who perform the work of an organization to achieve that organization's goals.

Effective Team Building

Effective teams are the key to the accomplishment of all work. By the year 2000, it is projected that most organizations will be more decentralized and workers will be broken up into special work units, where they have responsibility for all functions relating to their work.

These small teams will be autonomous for work products, including outcomes and even budget accountability. The cultures of some progressive companies are already structuring their work environments to facilitate this goal.

The Nurse Manager's Role With the Team

You manage a nursing unit where all work is accomplished by your team. Your team-building role provides a unique opportunity to develop staff, problem solve, and meet the care needs of patients. The leader of any team determines the style of the team. Your most important and ongoing roles are communicator and being a role model. This is ensured through the following activities:

TIPS FOR MANAGING A SUCCESSFUL TEAM

✔ Manage in a way that demonstrates respect to staff, peers, and others

✔ Remind staff of the task at hand

✔ Respect the team for their professional skills and knowledge

✔ Project self-confidence

✔ Show enthusiasm

✔ Listen and problem solve

✔ Be flexible

✔ Provide support

✔ Be organized

✔ Continually use your human relation skills

✔ Create an atmosphere of cooperation and collaboration

✔ Keep the team on track and focused

✔ Recognize staff

✔ Give feedback

✔ Share common goals

✔ Give staff accountability and responsibility

✔ Delegate effectively

✔ Manage with a clear vision of where you are going; share it often

✔ Allow staff to take risks

✔ Provide encouragement and feedback

✔ Clarify assignments when needed

✔ Reward staff for work well done

✔ Create and nurture rapport

✔ Follow up on problems

✔ Empower staff

✔ Write about your team and their accomplishments in memos, newsletters, professional journals, and local papers

✔ Be there to provide help when needed

✔ Lead a well balanced life

✔ Create an ego-enhancing environment

✔ Foster a cooperative environment

✔ Demonstrate retention-directed management skills

✔ Choose new team members effectively

✔ Keep lines of communication open

✔ Recognize individual nurse's contributions

✔ Communicate to your supervisor the work accomplished by your team

✔ Maintain and use your sense of humor

✔ Share patient evaluation feedback with staff

✔ Remove obstacles to work completion

✔ Let go of owning all problems and solutions once you have delegated the work

✔ Ask for suggestions on better ways to do things

✔ Ask "What can I do to help you get your work done more effectively?"

Managers can create a motivating environment that empowers their nursing staffs. An environment where communications are open, where the manager listens, and where staff feel they have input and influence in decisions enables nurses to be committed. The team leader or manager must be trustworthy, honest, have good active listening skills, and communicate with the staff frequently about the achievement of the unit's and department's goals.

THE TEAM MEMBERS

Numerous categories have been used in labeling types of team members. Examples include natural leaders, initiators, motivators, loyalists, and other various types that contribute to a team's make up. In fact, labeling team members as types may be counterproductive. However, each of us may exhibit these characteristics in different situations.

The best groups function effectively when they have input into the methods to be used in reaching the defined goal. It has been said that the true test of effective management is how well the group functions when the manager is not present. Therefore use your staff's natural skills and abilities. We all do best in tasks that we enjoy. So, when possible, let staff members choose assignments or tasks they want to perform. These roles can be clear at the onset. For example, delegate organizational responsibilities to a particularly well organized staff member. He or she can remind you of the time, take minutes of meetings, or reorganize an ineffective process through to resolution with input from other involved peer nurses.

Team Problems

All teams or staffs can have problems at one time or another. These problems can range in scope and significance and can affect the functioning of the unit as a whole. These problems can include the following symptoms.

- Cliques
- Increased errors or mistakes
- Isolation of new staff members
- Increased complaints
- "We" versus "they" feelings
- Scapegoating of specific staff member(s)
- Negative comments from peers or your manager
- Decreased productivity
- Silence
- Failure to share needed information among team members

When problem trends are identified, self-evaluation is indicated. Is the manager doing anything to increase the conflict? An example could be a reward system that reinforces undesirable behaviors. Does the staff feel or perceive that there are favorites who get better assignments or more staff education days than do others? For example, if one staff member goes to lunch with you, rotate this opportunity with all your staff. Certain behaviors or personalities can sometimes lead to conflict. The effective resolution of conflict is one of the responsibilities of all managers.

CONFLICT

It is important that the nurse manager remember that not all conflict needs intervention. Welcome the existence of differences in your work setting. Much has been written on conflict management and individual styles for conflict resolution. It is thought that we all use different styles in different situations, though we may have a favorite style. Use the presence of conflict as a possible indicator of the need for change or problem solving. Conflict can be a strong motivator.

Your Role in Conflict Resolution Between Staff Team Members

The following tips can help facilitate effective conflict resolution. Two traits are needed for effective conflict resolution: (1) trust, and (2) rationality.

TIPS FOR RESOLVING CONFLICTS

✔ Know that conflict is inevitable and not all conflict is destructive.

✔ Always work toward helping staff members settle differences themselves.

✔ View yourself not as a parent but as an objective observer only.

✔ Validate that you will not take sides.

✔ Be objective.

✔ Support harmony and resolution.

✔ Verbalize that staff members need to talk to each other and that you trust their problem solving skills.

✔ Listen with understanding, not judgement.

✔ Clarify the issue only when necessary.

✔ Do not criticize or deny feelings such as anger or fear.

✔ Focus on maintaining the relationship between the conflicting parties.

✔ Create a problem-solving atmosphere.

✔ Offer your office space for a limited time for this discussion, when appropriate.

✔ Be able to identify a chronically complaining employee. This is important because such behavior can contribute to a depressing tone for the entire work environment.

WHAT TO DO WHEN RESOLVING COMPLAINTS

✔ Listen to the complaint but set limits if it continues.

✔ Ask for the recommended solutions to the listed complaint.

✔ Work on the development of problem-solving skills for the staff members involved.

SUMMARY

In conclusion, interpersonal skills important to the nurse manager include a variety of overlapping traits, activities, and attitudes.

The successful manager is open and supportive of staff, truly seeing them behaviorally as valuable resources. Constant communication, which is well planned, executed, and validated, combined with real caring and investment in staff, creates an environment that fosters motivation, retention, and success.

The successful use of problem-solving skills ensures that the feelings and energy generated by conflict is directed toward creative resolution. This approach welcomes the uniqueness of all individuals and is potentially growth enhancing for individuals and teams.

REFERENCES

1. Lancaster J: Creating a climate for excellence, *J Nurs Adm* pp 16, January 1985.
2. Kramer M, Schmalenberg C: Job satisfaction and retention, *Nurs 91* 21:51, 1991.
3. Swansburg RC: *Management and leadership for nurse managers,* Boston, 1990, Jones & Bartlett.
4. Horsley J: When to tattle on physician's misconduct, *RN* 4(12):17, 1978. In Luquire R: Nursing risk management, *Nurs Manage* 20:56, 1989.
5. The National Joint Practice Commission: *The definition of joint or collaborative practice,* statement 4, September 1977.

CHAPTER 5

Day-to-Day Operations

Margaret A. Powers
T. M. Marrelli

It has been said that "managing makes a manager." However, it does help to have some information about the nursing manager's day-to-day duties and responsibilities before being faced with carrying them out.

Day-to-day operations are the core of the nurse manager's activities. Staffing and scheduling personnel, delivering nursing care through a nursing care delivery model, and meetings (including leading staff meetings and supporting patient care conferences) are all activities that are vital to the day-to-day functioning of a nursing unit or area. Information about these subjects as well as others relating to the day-to-day operation of a nursing unit or area are discussed in this chapter.

Intertwined with these subjects are the JCAHO standards, the ever-present need to be cost-effective and efficient, and the quest for positive patient outcome and high patient satisfaction. All these are considered while working to promote the professionalism and satisfaction of the nursing staff.

NURSING CARE DELIVERY SYSTEMS

New nurse managers need to understand the various types of nursing care delivery systems (NCDSs), the strengths and weaknesses of each, and their unique value in their own setting. In fact, Manthey[1] feels that of all areas of technical knowledge required to understand unit operations, nursing care delivery system options, including work structure, are the most important area to know.

A NCDS is the way in which nursing care is provided to the patient or, according to Wake,[2] is "an interacting set of structural ele-

91

TABLE 5-1   Frequency of Use of Nursing Care Delivery Systems

Type	Percentage
Team nursing	53.3
Total patient care	47.3
Primary nursing	32.1
Modular nursing	19.3
Functional nursing	13.6
Case management	5.7

The American Hospital Association's Center for Nursing: *1989 Hospital nursing personnel survey,* Chicago, 1989, The AHA.

ments which control the way care is provided." Manthey[3] says that a delivery system has to answer five questions:

1. Who is responsible for making decisions about patient care?
2. How long do that person's decisions remain in effect?
3. How is the work distributed among staff members—by task or by patient?
4. How is patient care communication handled?
5. How is the whole unit managed?

The six major NCDSs used across the country and their frequency of usage, based on a 1989 survey by the American Hospital Association's Center for Nursing, are noted in Table 5-1.[4]

Team Nursing

Team nursing is an NCDS that uses an RN as a team leader to lead a group of nursing staff, which may include other RNs, LPNs, or nursing assistants, to care for a group of patients together. Sherman[5] identifies a basic belief of team nursing—team members of varying skill levels can contribute to patient-centered nursing care if their activities are coordinated by a professional nurse.

The team leader is responsible for assessing the patients' needs, planning the care, and delegating tasks to the other members of the team based on their skills and abilities and within the scope of their job description. In addition, the team leader evaluates the care given and revises the plan of care as necessary.

The key to sucessful team nursing is communication among team members and with the patient and family. This is usually facilitated with the nursing care conference or team conference, which is held to coordinate care and to gain input from all the team members. Care can be evaluated from everyone's perspective and care plans developed and modified if necessary.

Proposed strengths of the team nursing system are efficiency and lower costs as compared with the total patient care and primary nursing systems, as well as making use of varying levels of nursing personnel. Theoretically, an esprit de corps develops among team members as they work together.

Negatives include a lack of accountability (because everyone is accountable) and the costs associated with the need for daily conference time. From the patient's point of view, several caregivers are involved with care rather than just one person. This results in a task-orientation versus total patient care approach, which increases fragmentation of care.

Total Patient Care

Total patient care is an NCDS in which the RN or LPN is given the assignment of planning, organizing, and giving care to a group of patients for a particular shift. The RN supervising the LPN may perform some assessment and planning activities on the LPN's assigned patients, but generally most care is performed by the nurse assigned.

Strengths of the total patient care system are fewer caregivers for the patient and theoretically a better knowledge of the patient by the assigned nurse because the numbers of assigned patients are less than with team nursing.

Weaknesses of the system are a greater cost as compared with the team nursing system and a possible lack of continuity and accountability—each nurse is assigned for only her shift, and some aspects of care for the patient may be overlooked or neglected.

Primary Nursing

Primary nursing is an NCDS in which the RN, called a primary nurse, is given an assignment of planning and organizing all care for a group of patients for the total hospitalization of those patients, 24 hours a day. The primary nurse may also give the care but may delegate particular aspects. When the primary nurse is not on duty, an associate nurse cares for patients using the plan set forth by the primary nurse.

Primary nursing provides a nurse who has accountability for outcomes of care and care planning and documentation. Usually there is high patient satisfaction, continuity of care, and care of a high quality. Of course primary nursing is only as good as the primary nurse, and it is considered more costly than team or functional nursing because it usually relies on a larger number of RNs.

Modular Nursing

Modular nursing is an NCDS in which an RN is assigned the nursing care for a group of patients, generally grouped geographically, along with another caregiver (either an LPN or an unlicensed staff member). It is a form of team nursing in principle but uses smaller teams. It provides closer monitoring of care than does team nursing and uses fewer RNs than the primary nursing system. It is less costly than primary nursing and can use other types of caregivers. It is, however, less efficient and costs more than team nursing.

Functional Nursing

Functional nursing is an NCDS in which each caregiver is given a task to perform within the scope of her abilities and job description for all the patients on a unit. The patient thus sees a number of caregivers, each an expert in her particular task (similar to an assembly line.) One nurse gives medications and another gives treatments; an aide changes linen, and so on.

It is considered the most efficient and least costly form of care, requiring fewer RNs. It takes advantage of differing skill levels.

However, from the patient's perspective, functional nursing focuses more on tasks rather than meeting the patient's needs with multiple caregivers, who may not see the patient as a whole. From the staff's point of view, boredom may result from performing repetitious activities.

Case Management

Case management is a form of primary nursing whereby the RN who is the case manager is responsible for managing the nursing care of a group of patients across all units during that hospitalization. Protocols are developed by the health care team to achieve clinical outcomes within prescribed time frames.

The case management NCDS has all the advantages of primary nursing. Although primary nursing is considered costly, the emphasis on protocols and meeting outcomes within time frames may help to save money in the long run because of reduction in lengths of stay. It also promotes nursing professionalism and collegiality with other disciplines.

Facilities across the country have adopted one or more of the NCDSs described. Most have modified the original system as proposed and tailored it to meet the needs of their settings and the availability of staff. Keep in mind that any NCDS can be used with any skill level and mix of staff. Factors that influence which model is chosen include:

- The values and philosophy of the facility, especially those of the nursing department
- The numbers and quality of available nursing personnel
- Consumer demands
- Competition in the marketplace
- The retention status of staff members
- Financial status of the institution or how much money is available to spend on salaries for staff members

In 1989, a survey was done by Wake[2] that asked for the status of, among other things, patient assignment in 1986 and 1989 and projections for 1992. Results showed that although team nursing and primary nursing NCDSs increased from 1986 to 1989, the case management system was projected by far to be the NCDS of choice by 1992. In fact, the case management system is not yet the NCDS of choice, but it undoubtedly will be in the near future. Obviously, we see that the models of nursing care delivery are evolving.

Professionally Advanced Care Team Model

Several NCDSs have been successfully implemented that may be of some interest. The Professionally Advanced Care Team model (ProACT) was developed through the work redesign process. This NCDS delineates two RN roles, the primary nurse and the clinical care manager. The primary nurse manages primary patients and delegates care giving to LPNs, associate nurses, and nursing assistants. The clinical care manager manages the entire hospital stay of a caseload of patients and ensures outcomes are met, much like the case manager. In addition, this model features unit-based nonclinical support personnel who function to relieve the nursing staff of nonnursing duties.

Partners in Practice

A form of primary nursing (or modular nursing) is partners in practice, which uses nurse extenders coupled with an RN to form a "partnership" to care for a group of patients together. The RN and nurse helper work the same schedule on the same shift to give care to patients. The RN assesses and plans care and delegates selected activities to the nurse extender.

Coprimary Nursing

Coprimary nursing is an NCDS whereby two nurses function together as one to be the primary nurse. They work the same shift on differing days to provide continuity. This system was developed originally in the critical care setting to help deal with the fragmentation of 12-hour shifts.

Patient-Centered Care

Many hospitals across the country have begun to restructure delivery systems to become more patient-oriented as opposed to hospital-oriented. Services are being organized around meeting the individual needs of the patient. This change in focus involves an analysis and redefinition of all activities involved with patients, a work redesign. It involves all departments that deal with the patient, including the nursing department, and is truly multidisciplinary in approach.

After work redesign is implemented, often "multipurpose" roles are created to perform ancillary tasks and procedures for patients that were formerly done in other departments, such as the admission registration process in admissions, a phlebotomy in the laboratory, or an electrocardiogram (ECG) in the cardiology department. Often these activities are all carried out in the patient's room by one person, who may be teamed with an RN. Many systems have the nurse manager or staff nurses supervising these individuals.

Forces driving the restructuring efforts are customer service concerns and consumer demands, quality and efficiency needs, the shortage of RNs, and the need to reduce costs.

As more and more institutions are restructuring care, we are likely to see other innovations in NCDSs emerge.

Evaluation of the Nursing Care Delivery System

One role of the new nurse manager is to analyze the current NCDS for adequacy. The following questions should be posed:

- Are patient outcomes being achieved in a timely, cost-effective manner?
- Are patients and families satisfied with care?
- Are physicians and other health team members satisfied with the care?

Information on how to conduct an in-depth analysis of an NCDS is available in *Nursing Assignment Patterns User's Manual* by Munson et al.[6] Piltz-Kirkby[7] discusses her experience using the tool on a rehabilitation unit. How to gather information on patient characteristics, nursing resources, and organizational support is described, as well as a way to analyze the data gathered. An informed decision can then be made to keep or change the NCDS.

The JCAHO standards do not specifically dictate which type of NCDS a facility should adopt. They do address roles of the nursing staff and the mechanism used to assign staff members. Standards that are relevant to NCDSs are noted in the box on p. 98.[8]

PROFESSIONAL PRACTICE MODELS

Although the NCDSs previously described address assignment of patients and roles of nursing personnel, they do not identify underlying professional practice issues such as autonomy in professional decision making, budgeting of time for care activities, and nursing practice growth and development. Professional practice models do address these issues.

Shared Governance

Many facilities have adopted some sort of shared governance model within nursing. Shared governance is an organizational model that gives staff the authority for decisions, autonomy to make those decisions, and control over the implementation and outcomes of the decisions. Authority and accountability are shared between and among all the staff and the organization as partners.[9] Various models are in practice, but generally, councils or cabinets of staff nurses are developed, with staff members serving in leadership roles and management advising and supporting. By-laws are developed that guide

---

JCAHO STANDARDS RELATED TO NURSING CARE DELIVERY SYSTEMS

NC.1 Patients receive nursing care based on a documented assessment of their needs.

 NC.1.1 Each patient's need for nursing care related to his/her admission is assessed by a registered nurse.

  NC.1.1.2 Aspects of data collection may be delegated by the registered nurse.

  NC.1.3.2 Nursing staff members collaborate, as appropriate, with physicians and other clinical disciplines in making decisions regarding each patient's need for nursing care.

 NC.3.4 Policies and procedures describe the mechanism used to assign nursing staff members to meet patient care needs.

  NC3.4.1 There are sufficient qualified nursing staff members to meet the nursing care needs of patients throughout the hospital.

   NC.3.4.1.1 The criteria for employment, deployment, and assignment of nursing staff members are approved by the nursing executive.

 NC.4.1 The plan for nurse staffing and the provision of nursing care are reviewed in detail on an annual basis and receive periodic attention as warranted by changing patient care needs and outcomes.

  NC.4.1.1 Registered nurses prescribe, delegate, and coordinate the nursing care throughout the hospital.

Reprinted with permission from *Accreditation manual for hospitals,* 1992 ed, Oakbrook Terrace, Ill, Joint Commission on Accreditation of Healthcare Organizations.

the function of the nursing department. Nursing practice is defined by the staff through their council, and they, not the nurse manager, are accountable for the level of that practice. Likewise, staff members are accountable for all quality improvement and related activities. Continuing development and competency are determined by the staff council as well.

Compensation Innovation

Other concepts that have been integrated into some professional practice models are changes in compensation. Salaried nursing staff[10] and gain sharing[11] have been successfully implemented. The idea of "group-practices" has emerged; it is similar to the physician model. A group of nurses contracts to care for a group of patients for a specified period.[12]

The role of the nurse manager in the new practice models changes dramatically from the traditional one of "supervisor." The manager role is one of support and facilitation, ensuring that proper resources are available to the staff of her unit or area so they can do their jobs. Although it takes time to change philosophy, the result is a staff who have control over their practice, practice in a professional manner, and are more fulfilled and satisfied.

PATIENT CLASSIFICATION

A comprehensive staffing system comprises a patient classification system or acuity system, a master staffing plan, a scheduling plan, a position control plan, a budget, and reports that provide feedback to the manager on all components.

Patient classification is defined as "the categorization or grouping of patients according to an assessment of their nursing care requirements over a specified period of time."[13] It is seen as an objective and structured process to use in determining and allocating staff for patient care. In other words, patients are classified based on the projected number of nursing hours required to provide care. It can also be used as a measure of productivity and to help achieve compliance with JCAHO standards. With increasing concerns about scarce resources, cost, and efficiency, patient classification systems can assist with appropriate allocation of resources to meet patient needs and provide justification as necessary for the decisions made.

Although the JCAHO do not specifically mention patient classification tools or systems in their standards, they discuss the need for "nurse staffing plans for each unit which define the number and mix of nursing personnel in accordance with current patient care needs." They also state "staffing schedules are reviewed and adjusted as necessary to meet defined patient needs and unusual occurrences."[8]

These standards imply the use of some type of patient classification system. Patient classification can also be used to determine the cost of and bill for nursing services.

The patient classification process generally has two parts: (1) the actual classification procedure itself (using a tool), and (2) the quantification of the hours needed for the nursing care or staffing standards determined for each care category. In other words, for each category of care needed, from those patients needing the lowest amounts of nursing care to those requiring the most, an average number of nursing care hours is determined. Usually the tools are transferrable among facilities with similar groups of patients, but the staffing standards are not because of variations such as strength of support services, environmental factors such as unit or area layout, differences in philosophy including type of NCDS, differences in medical treatment, and levels and experience of nursing staff. Either work-sampling studies measuring indirect and direct care time or estimation procedures through trial and error can be performed to establish staffing standards for a tool borrowed from another facility.

Literally hundreds of patient classification systems are in use across the country. Some were developed specifically for a particular institution, and others were purchased from vendors. In a recent study, Nagaprasanna[14] found that a patient classification system is applicable to all types of nursing delivery systems. He also noted that internally developed systems were the most frequent type used, with four categories of patient acuity being the most common number of categories. Most facilities classify patients daily, and most systems are computerized, not manual. He found that the ease of classification is the highest rated factor in selecting a patient classification system.

The new nurse manager should become thoroughly familiar with the facility's system. Usually the system is managed by a person in the organization who assisted with its development and implementation, and this is the person to seek out to explain the system. Questions to ask include the following.

TIPS ON WHAT TO ASK ABOUT CLASSIFICATION SYSTEMS

✔ **Is the patient classification tool based on prototype evaluation or on factor-analysis evaluation?** (Prototypes are broad descriptions of three or four levels, and the patient is compared to the levels and placed in the one that most closely matches his or her description. Factor-analysis is based on a list of critical indicators that, when summed up, indicate a patient category.)

✔ **What is the process by which the tool is used by the nursing staff?** It is essential to know each and every step. As issues arise, an awareness of where "things can go wrong" is helpful in solving problems with the system.

✔ **How is the system maintained and monitored? What is the role of the manager?** You need to know what orientation and ongoing educational programs for staff are available as relates to the system. Reliability checks are usually built into the system. Reliability means consistency between raters. Achieving agreement of at least 90% is generally considered acceptable.[13]

Validity monitoring refers to whether the system actually measures what it is supposed to measure. Sometimes surveys of the staff are done or actual time-motion studies are conducted to reaffirm the system.

✔ **How are data generated by the system interpreted? What should be done with data once they are interpreted?** Obviously the manager must understand what the data mean and then how they can be used as *aids* to staff the unit. Most systems compile and report an acuity number that is the sum of all patients' levels. They then predict the numbers of staff needed on the following shifts.

✔ **What exactly is patient classification used for in the facility? Only for staffing on a daily basis? For the yearly budget? For productivity? For assignments? For placement of patients on units? For determining costs of patient services?**

✔ **What are the current problems with the system?** The nurse manager should also ask this question of the staff. Sometimes there are problems with "acuity creep," or gradually rising acuity levels. Usually it is a managerial responsibility to identify and work at resolving problems related to the system.

Two final points must be made concerning patient classification. First, the manager should understand that a high activity level in the unit or area and the acuity level of patients are not necessarily one and the same. Other causes exist that influence activity levels besides higher acuity levels, including factors such as experience and competency of the staff and presence and quality of support services at the unit level. Second, patient classification data are used as *supports* for decision making. They never take the place of nurse manager judgement, nor should they ever be taken as facts not to be questioned. Despite millions of dollars expended to find the perfect system, no such thing exists. Keep that in mind.

SCHEDULING AND STAFFING

One of the activities that consumes the most time available to managers is scheduling and staffing. In a 1990 survey of nurse managers by the American Organization of Nurse Executives (AONE),[15]

TABLE 5-2   Types of Scheduling Patterns

Pattern	Comments
8-hour/5-day week	Still the predominant pattern. Allows for a 30 minute meal break and a 30 minute overlap time if used for 24 hours.
10-hour/4-day week	Gives an opportunity for longer overlaps during activity times, meetings, or educational sessions. Allows the staff an extra day off each week.
10-hour/7-day week	Staff works 7 days on and has 7 days off. Gives better continuity and periods of time off, but fatigue has been reported by the end of the work week.
Baylor plan	Staff member works only on weekends and either works 2 days with 12-hour shifts and is paid for 36 hours, or 2 nights and is paid for 40 hours.
12-hour/3-day week	Gives better continuity over the course of the shift but not over the week. Allows staff 4 days off during week.

it was found that 11.1% of their time was spent on this activity. Not only time but concern and worry also are often hallmarks of this activity because the manager is ultimately responsible to see that the facility is staffed appropriately. There can be legal ramifications if staffing is not appropriate.

Nursing staff are very concerned about scheduling and staffing. In fact, the American Journal of Nursing[16] conducted a survey of its readers in 1987 and found that a "desired work schedule" was 1 of the 10 most important items that influenced decisions on whether to stay in nursing. Another top item was "having an adequate nurse/patient ratio," which again relates to scheduling and staffing. Clearly these two areas affect nurse retention, so sensibly, the new manager should be aware of scheduling and staffing practices and options.

Scheduling Patterns and Options

In the past 20 years, various types of scheduling practices and options have been developed over and above the traditional 8-hour-a-day, 5-day-a-week schedule. Several of the most prevalent patterns are noted in Table 5-2.

Almost every conceivable combination of shifts and days has been tried somewhere in the quest to find schedules that fit into every nurse's lifestyle, still meet patient care needs, and yet fit within the personnel budget and unit staffing model.

Cyclical schedules lend a degree of predictability to a staff member's schedule by using a pattern that is repeated consistently over a certain number of weeks.

Rotating shifts or permanent shifts for staff members are often an issue. Rotating shifts helps to share the burden of the less popular shifts and increases cooperation between shifts, but it does cause stress, depending on how often the rotation is done. Permanent shifts better meet staff members' needs, but a problem usually arises because most nurses want the popular daytime shift. In that case, seniority often determines who gets which shift. Rifts between shifts may happen with greater frequency with permanent shifts than with rotation shifts.

Control of staffing can be highly centralized, which may be more efficient and fair, or it can be decentralized, to the manager level or even down to the staff level, better meeting staff members' own individual needs.

Centralized scheduling can apply facility staffing and scheduling policies fairly throughout nursing, so no one individual or group gets preferential treatment. It is easier to use float or per diem staff to fill in empty shift spots with centralization. Computerization can be used with centralized scheduling. Data are entered on staff members' preferences and on facility policies and procedures regarding staffing and scheduling. Unit staffing patterns are identified, and patient classification data is entered. No doubt the advantages of computer scheduling include an easy-to-read schedule, fairness and consistency, and less time spent by the manager doing the schedule. However, centralized scheduling does set up a "we" versus "they" situation. Staff members may not feel any obligation to solve problems in the process of staffing and scheduling because it is not their job, but the job of the central staffing and scheduling office. They may feel that centralized scheduling lacks individual attention and also feel that the schedule does not meet their needs.

Decentralized scheduling can be done by the manager or the staff. If the nurse manager does the schedule, she often becomes an expert very quickly. She best knows the needs of the unit and of the staff, if the staff communicate with her. It does take the manager large amounts of time to produce a schedule, especially if a variety of scheduling options are available to the staff. One significant problem with the manager creating the schedule is that some staff members may perceive that others get favored treatment. Although this may or may not be true, it is very easy for the manager to misguidedly use scheduling as a reward-and-punishment system.

Self-scheduling by staff is being adopted by more and more facilities. Ringl and Dotson[17] describe it as a "process by which nurses collectively develop and implement the monthly work schedule." Criteria are mutually agreed on by the work group and applied. Peers can negotiate and trade within the guidelines. Often an individual staff nurse or scheduling committee oversee(s) the process, a position which may be rotated among every member of the work group. The manager usually works with the group, especially when beginning the process. Although implementation of self-scheduling is not without problems, the process usually goes more smoothly the longer it is in place. Most staff members do not want to give it up once they have worked with it. It is said to increase job satisfaction, increase autonomy and control, and decrease turnover and absenteeism.[17]

Staffing

Despite the best scheduling efforts, staffing disasters do occur. Nurse managers should be aware of the options available to deal with these crises and of the fact that everyone has them at one time or another, to a greater or lesser extent.

Sick calls are notorious for causing the manager headaches. They can be handled in a variety of ways, depending on the options available in your facility.

TIPS FOR HANDLING AN UNCOVERED SHIFT

✔ Use a float, per diem, or agency nurse assistance

✔ Ask a part-time staff member to work the extra shift

✔ Ask a staff member to work for the person who is ill and cancel a subsequent shift later in the week

✔ Ask a staff member of the previous shift to stay over for either part of the shift or the whole shift

✔ Ask a staff member on the shift following the shift in question to come in for the whole shift or part of the shift

✔ Substitute one type of job classification for another, such as a nursing assistant for an RN or vice versa

✔ Do without anyone

✔ Work the shift yourself

There are pros and cons with each method used. One point to make about the final option is that new managers particularly often work the shift themselves because it is the easiest solution. Although it may initially solve the problem, working as a staff member herself by necessity leaves other parts of her job undone. This may ultimately hurt the staff more than it helps them. It is up to the manager to help the staff learn that each member has a job to do that is valuable and to get them to feel a responsibility to help with staffing as much as does the manager.

Sometimes, if the supply of staff cannot be obtained, the manager can meet the need by working from the other side of the equation; that is, by reducing the need for staffing by transferring patients, screening types of patients that enter the system and thereby lowering acuity, or by "closing" beds.

Particularly during periods of nursing shortages, the manager might experience high vacancies on the unit. Although the solutions identified on p. 104 for sick calls might help on an occasional basis, staff burnout will occur if they are used for prolonged periods. Using agency or traveling nurses has helped many facilities cope with vacancies until positions could be filled permanently. Closing, or "holding," beds also helps the situation. This practice, however, may decrease revenue for the facility if the patient goes elsewhere. The reasons for the vacancies and/or why positions cannot be filled should be thoroughly investigated and the causes fixed.

A master staffing plan (i.e., the guideline or plan by which the area is usually staffed) is usually developed for each area or unit. It is important for the manager to secure a copy of the plan and understand its components backwards and forwards. The components are the staffing pattern that gives the numbers and types of staff members to schedule on each shift and the numbers and types of staff members to hire to fulfill the pattern.

The design of the staffing pattern is based on a standard or statistic determined by the facility. That statistic will vary from facility to facility and might include factors such as patient acuity level and associated required hours of nursing care, census, numbers of procedures, and so on. Table 5-3 displays a staffing pattern for a 33-bed general surgical unit. The statistics which determined this pattern were patient acuity with associated hours of nursing care and patient census. Remember that this pattern is built on *averages*, usually identified from historical data. As you know, anything can happen, in which case deviations will occur from the pattern.

TABLE 5-3   Example of Master Staffing Pattern

33-bed capacity	Su	M	Tu	W	Th	F	Sa	
DAY SHIFT								
RN	4	5	5	6	6	5	4	35
LPN	1	2	2	2	2	2	1	12
AIDE	2	2	3	3	3	3	2	18
TOTAL	7	9	10	11	11	10	7	65
EVENING SHIFT								
RN	4	5	5	5	5	5	4	33
LPN	1	1	1	1	1	1	1	7
AIDE	1	1	1	1	1	1	1	7
TOTAL	6	7	7	7	7	7	6	47
NIGHT SHIFT								
RN	3	4	4	4	4	4	3	26
LPN	0	0	0	0	0	0	0	0
AIDE	1	1	1	1	1	1	1	7
TOTAL	4	5	5	5	5	5	4	33
TOTAL NURSING HRS	136	168	176	184	184	176	136	165.7 (average)
AVERAGE CENSUS	25	30.5	32	32.8	32.8	32	25	29.9 (average)
HOURS OF CARE	5.40	5.50	5.50	5.60	5.60	5.50	5.40	5.54 (average)
AVERAGE ACUITY	2.20	2.30	2.40	2.45	2.45	2.40	2.30	2.37 (average)

The pattern displayed indicates the number and type of staff members that should be routinely scheduled based on an average daily census and acuity score, which dictates the hours of nursing care desired. Decisions were made about the distribution of staff members by job category based on patient needs and work requirements.

The pattern should be reviewed periodically to see if staffing practices need to be changed based on statistical increases or decreases or on other factors such as the strength of support departments or changes in patient mix or flow.

From such staffing pattern is built a full-time equivalent (FTE) budget to which nonproductive hours are added, such as vacation, holiday, and sick hours and staff development time. An FTE is equal to 2080 hours worked per year (i.e., what a person would work if 40 hours a week, 52 weeks a year were spent working). The budget is then translated into positions which are designated full-time or part-time, and it is used as a basis to hire personnel.

It is a good idea to share the staffing pattern with staff members so they understand how it was developed and can assist in supporting it.

LIABILITY CONCERNED WITH STAFFING

On a daily basis, the nurse manager often faces the problem of trying to staff the area or unit with dwindling resources while still maintaining a standard of nursing care. Indeed, the manager's job description usually states something like, "is accountable for staffing the unit on a 24-hour basis." Questions may arise as to the liability of the nurse manager in relation to unsafe staffing levels; to float, registry, or agency nurse errors; to staff refusal to accept a unit or float assignment; and possibly to nurses walking off the job. As background for addressing these issues, the nurse manager should become familiar with the facility's rules, regulations, policies, and procedures concerned with staffing, floating, and overtime. They will help direct decisions that must be made when problems arise. If the day comes when all options to cover an unsafe staffing situation have been tried to no avail, the next step is to communicate the inadequate staffing situation to the supervisor.[18] The guiding principle is that of reasonableness. If the nurse manager has done everything possible to solve the problem and has communicated that fact to the appropriate persons, then she is most likely absolved of liability for the situation. The situation should be documented in a report, dated and signed, and sent to the manager's supervisor. The write-up should be factual and describe what effect the situation may have on patient care.

The use of float, registry, or agency nurses is one way some facilities are coping with the nursing shortage in general or with occasional staffing deficiencies. Is the nurse manager liable for their actions? According to Fiesta,[19] the manager may be placed in secondary liability for these nurses. These nurses must be screened and oriented as is the regular staff. Baillie et al,[20] regarding float nurses, said, "Regardless, before floating any nurse, supervisors should determine her level of knowledge, the skills necessary, and functions required in the new assignment and provide adequate orientation."

With agency nurses, the manager should try to assign them to low-risk situations and ensure that the patients realize the nurse is an agency nurse. If any question arises as to competency, the manager has a duty to report that, in writing, back to the agency. Of course, the nurse manager should follow the facility's standard operating procedures regarding communication with the agency.

What if a staff nurse refuses an assignment or threatens to walk off the job? It is wise not to react too quickly to the situation. Often the refusal or threat results from fear or feeling unprepared. The manager should sit down and unemotionally discuss the situation with the nurse. Find out what would make the nurse accept the situation and then attempt to remedy the problem if it seems reasonable. If it does not seem reasonable and if after talking the situation is not resolved, the manager should be sure the nurse has been given a clear and direct order that is not misinterpreted as a suggestion or request or as advice. The nurse should be queried as to whether the order is understood and is clear and whether she is refusing to do the order. The manager may want to forewarn the nurse of possible consequences if the order is refused. These consequences could be disciplinary action and perhaps even being fired, depending on the facility's personnel policies and practices.

CREDENTIALING

Recently an increasing focus has been placed on credentialing nursing staff. This may have resulted in part from the changes in the JCAHO nursing standards, which were implemented in 1991. Credentialing encompasses licensure, accreditation, certification, and academic degrees.[21] The nursing manager usually has a role to play in ensuring that the process is implemented and that the nurses practicing in her area are competent. Credentialing came about because it benefits and protects the patient by ensuring that the nurse has certain minimum skills and abilities. A nursing license ensures these skills and abilities on entry into practice but *does not guarantee ongoing competency*. With medical and nursing practice changing so rapidly, additional credentialing activities need to be added to licensure to ensure ongoing competency.

During the interview, the nurse manager discusses grades, degrees, and experience with the potential new employee. Licensure is checked, and a copy is often made and inserted into the personnel file if the nurse is hired. Other information on courses attended may be obtained.

Usually during an orientation period, performance standards are met by the orientee. A skills inventory is completed after satisfactory demonstration of skills such as patient assessment, care planning, or medication administration, and this is maintained in the personnel record of an individual nurse. This inventory needs to be dated and signed. The skills inventory, or orientation checklist, provides legal documentation of professional skills competency. Additional specialty courses may be completed and tests taken that show mastery of the material (e.g., fetal monitoring or group therapy facilitation). The nurse manager's role is to ensure that this process happens through to filing the results. Often the skills inventory will be distributed, explained, and even completed, but never make it to the personnel record.

Remedial study may need to be undertaken if deficiencies are identified through critical incidents. It may be up to the manager to see that a plan is formulated with the individual nurse to correct deficiencies and attain the necessary skills and knowledge.

One area that is very difficult to develop and implement in credentialing is maintaining competence and ensuring that current staff members have the knowledge and ability to carry out selected clinical tasks. Recently the JCAHO has emphasized this area by stating, "All members of the nursing staff are competent to fulfill their assigned responsibilities."[8] JCAHO asserted that not only should competence be assessed on initial employment and orientation, but that ongoing competence assessment and educational activities are necessary. Usually the facility decides what is to be assessed and how often assessment will occur. For instance, in a coronary care unit, the proficiency of defibrillation may be assessed every year by observation. Sometimes self-learning modules that include testing at the end might be used.

It is important that the nursing staff understand why their competence is being checked and that they participate in the determination and development of the plan for ensuring competency.

Another aspect of credentialing is external certification. Almost every nursing specialty organization has a mechanism for certification. A test is taken and, in some cases, proof is required for a certain amount and type of clinical experience. Attainment of certification ensures a certain level of knowledge. For more information on certification, please refer to Chapter 13.

Many facilities promote external certification by reimbursing nurses or by making it part of the requirements for a higher level within a clinical ladder system. Review courses associated with particular tests are often given in the facility. Manager support of external certification helps the staff pursue this additional level of professional expertise.

MEETINGS

All organizations hold meetings of one type or another, health care institutions being no exception. Indeed, because the nature of the business usually encompasses 24 hours a day, 7 days a week, with a multitude of various departments and disciplines participating, the need for meetings may even be higher than in the industrial or general business sector.

New nurse managers must acquire the skills for either leading or helping others to lead meetings if the managers are to function at an optimum level in today's modern health care institutions. Gone are the days when a manager issued a dictum without consulting others in the work group. Group problem-solving activities and planning for change with group consensus are common practices, and leaders are needed to make the meeting processes efficient and help ensure the best outcomes.

STAFF MEETINGS

In general, the most common meeting a new nurse manager will lead is the group staff meeting. Purposes of a staff meeting vary depending on the situation for which the meeting is called (Table 5-4). Identifying the purpose is important because that assists group members in knowing what is desired of them and gives the nurse manager some guidance on what leadership techniques to use.

Meetings are expensive when the salaries of all involved are analyzed. Thus some techniques can be used to make a meeting effi-

TABLE 5-4   Purposes of Staff Meetings and Leadership Techniques to Use

Purpose	Techniques
Giving information (manager to group)	• Be sure the group understands what has been told to them by soliciting questions, approval, criticism, and so on.
Receiving information (group to manager)	• Ask clear questions and listen. • Use a "round robin" technique to solicit information from less verbal group members.
Interactional (group and manager)	• Combination of above.
Problem solving/decision making	• Help group identify real problem. • Use brain-storming techniques for alternatives. • Get consensus of solution. • Ensure actions are assigned.

BEHAVIORS FOR LEADING EFFECTIVE MEETINGS

1. Prepare by drawing up an agenda well before the meeting, posting it, and allowing addition of items by the staff. Identify the purpose of the meeting.
2. Be sure all agenda items are necessary. Some might be better addressed in a memo, a message posted on the bulletin board, or dealt with on a one-to-one basis.
3. Start and end promptly. Keep on schedule. Close the discussion if necessary but be prepared to readdress unfinished business later.
4. Clarify and summarize discussions and/or decisions so the group is clear on outcomes. Lend structure to the discussion.
5. Ask vocal members to allow others to contribute. Encourage the less vocal members to talk.
6. Keep a neutral, friendly, and respectful attitude while leading. Thank everyone for attending.
7. If necessary, request that arguments, criticisms, and side conversations be held until after the meeting.
8. Set up an environment conducive to the meeting, including adequate ventilation, room temperature, and seating. Interruptions should be kept to a minimum.
9. Have all hand-outs available, including agenda.
10. Assure that minutes are taken.

---

cient and get its purpose accomplished. The box above describes behaviors for leading an effective meeting.

Attendees at the group staff meeting are usually chosen according to the philosophy of the organization and past practice. Options include meeting with just the members of a particular position, (i.e., RNs or nursing assistants); all staff members from a particular shift; or the total staff. There are pros and cons for each grouping. Small groups of 4 to 12 people seem to work best together. However, it is best to allow the group as a whole to decide who should attend the staff meetings. They should also determine the frequency, time(s) of the day, day(s) of the week, and length of the meeting.

The JCAHO has standards that have implications for group staff meetings. Standard NC.2.3 states that, "Nursing staff members participate in orientation, regularly scheduled staff meetings, and ongoing education designed to improve their competence." Standard NC.2.3.1 says, "Participation is documented."[8]

It is through documentation of the staff meetings (minutes), that evidence can be found that standards are being met. Thus it is vitally important for the staff meeting minutes to be accurate, specific, and detailed as to discussions, decisions, action plans, and so on.

Minutes should be retained on the unit for at least 3 years. However, the facility record retention policy should be followed in any case. The tips below describe important points to document in staff meeting minutes.

IMPORTANT POINTS TO DOCUMENT IN STAFF MEETING MINUTES

✔ Who did attend and who did not attend.

✔ Issues discussed and decisions regarding the issues, with an emphasis on those related to patient care.

✔ Quality improvement monitoring results should be presented with conclusions identified, recommendations by the group noted, and action plans listed. The process for evaluation should be identified by the group, highlighting the group's involvement in the process. When problems are corrected, this should be identified in the minutes.

✔ Any issues relating to patient care standards, standards of practice, or patient care delivery systems should be detailed, along with the resultant decisions and/or actions. Reports by staff representatives on committees should be documented.

Two issues frequently arise in relation to staff meetings that the new nurse manager must often address: (1) the lack of attendance at staff meetings, and (2) pay for attendance. In the former case, this is a problem the staff itself should address to determine the cause(s) and the solution. Absenteeism may be related to inconvenient times, inefficiently run meetings, or several other problems. Regarding the latter issue, most institutions have pay policies that outline whether staff members are paid for time spent at staff meetings when coming in on their own time. If not, a different policy would need to be developed by HR and/or Nursing Administration personnel because such a policy would affect the budget throughout the nursing department, if not the entire facility.

At times, the new nurse manager may lead other groups besides staff groups. These may include ad hoc groups formed to address issues or goals of the department or facility. The same principles identified earlier can be applied to leading these groups as well.

CLINICAL CONFERENCES

In today's fast-paced, complex, highly regulated health care environment, it is essential that patient care be administered efficiently so patient outcomes can be achieved as rapidly as possible. Clinical conferences help in this process by assisting in the coordination of care for the patient among all the disciplines involved. Duplication of effort and unnecessary confusion and frustration for the patient, family, and health care team can often be eliminated by holding a clinical conference.

Although the primary nurse or the RN most closely associated with the patient usually leads the conference, the new nurse manager definitely has a role to play in the process. Mahan[22] believes that the nurse manager suggests, encourages, validates, role models, and educates and is a resource person and quality control agent.

Various members of the health care team may participate, including the physician, social worker, utilization review nurse, pastoral care staff, therapists, dietician, home health nurse, and any others deemed necessary.

Often the family and even the patient participate in the conference as well. Once someone on the team, the patient, or the family decides a clinical conference is necessary, a leader is chosen, persons who should attend are identified, and a mutually accepted date and time are chosen. A conference room is procured. Arrangements may need to be made to cover the RN's assignment while she attends the conference. At the beginning of the conference, attendees are introduced, the purpose is highlighted, and the leader gives a brief overview of the patient's status, encouraging others to add additional data. Issues are identified, alternatives are discussed, and an action plan is formulated. Consensus is reached on follow-up and evaluation plans and the need for further meetings. The whole plan should be in the patient's record for easy access by all health care team members.

Documentation of the clinical conference should go beyond writing the action plan in the patient's record. Several JCAHO standards can be related to clinical conferences, and consistent documentation of attendees and the process and outcome of the conference will help

---

JCAHO STANDARDS RELATED TO CLINICAL CONFERENCES

NC.1 Patients receive nursing care based on a documented assessment of their needs.

NC.1.2 Each patient's assessment includes consideration of biophysical, psychosocial, environmental, self-care, educational, and discharge planning factors.

NC.1.3.1 The patient and/or significant other(s) are involved in the patient's care, as appropriate.

NC.1.3.2 Nursing staff members collaborate, as appropriate, with physicians and other clinical disciplines in making decisions regarding each patient's need for nursing care.

NC.1.3.3.1 In preparation for discharge, continuing care needs are assessed and referrals for such care are documented in the patient's medical record.

NC.1.3.4.5 The patient's response to, and the outcomes of, the care provided.

NC.1.3.4.6 The abilities of the patient and/or (as appropriate) his/her significant other(s) in managing continuing care needs after discharge.

Reprinted with permission from *Accreditation manual for hospitals*, 1992 ed, Oakbrook Terrace, Ill, Joint Commission on Accreditation of Healthcare Organizations.

demonstrate meeting these standards. The box above describes the standards relevant to clinical conferences.

ROUNDS IN THE CLINICAL AREA

Rounds made by the nurse manager in the areas where care is given can accomplish several things in a relatively short period. Making rounds gives information as to the performance of the staff because nursing care can be observed in practice and be compared with standards. Patient satisfaction with care received can be assessed by conversing with patients. Checks of the environment as to compliance with public health and safety standards can be done, and the area can be surveyed for aesthetic problems.

Although there is no hard-and-fast rule, daily rounds are suggested. Observations thus occur over a long period, and erroneous conclusions based on just a few observations can be avoided. Times of rounds during the day or night can be varied. Making notes as rounds are done assists in following up on issues that are identified. Staff members see the nurse manager as they work and may be more prone to bring up new issues when they see the manager. Stevens[23] feels that the presence of the manager on the nursing unit has the effect of decreasing the perceived distance between the employees and the manager. Also, the nursing staff feels that the manager knows what is going on, and this communicates authority.

Rather than putting patients on the spot with pointed questions concerning their perceptions of the quality of care, it is better to ask open-ended questions that might be less threatening, such as, "How is everything going? What is going on? or How are you doing?" If a patient's answer indicates the possibility of a problem, the manager can then focus the questioning further to get to the problem. Public health and safety standards should be reviewed by the manager by meeting with the person in the facility who is the most knowledgeable about them. One suggestion is to make a checklist from the standards that can be used during rounds to assess compliance. Aesthetic issues such as worn, broken, or tattered furnishings and building materials can be noted during rounds. The manager should view the unit or area as a patient or family might view it (similar to a hotel) and pass on a list of the deficiencies to the responsible department. Also, consider bringing in an objective person and asking for her or his aesthetic assessment and feedback for improvement.

Usually the list taken on rounds will have several items on it that the manager should plan to follow up.

PRIORITIZING DUTIES AND TIME MANAGEMENT

A manager's work is never done, and there is never enough time to do it all. Those concepts are difficult for a new nurse manager to accept. By the end of the day, as a staff nurse, most likely all one's tasks were finished. The nature of a manager's work is longer-term, and projects and activities may take more than just a day—often months, and occasionally, years—to complete. On a daily basis, managers must decide what activity or project takes precedence over another as they are faced with multiple and sometimes conflicting demands. How does the new manager prioritize her schedule?

Patients are important to a staff nurse, and they still are to a manager. Issues surrounding patients should be addressed promptly, such as patient complaints, staffing issues, or concerns related to supporting patient care. Top priority should be those issues which meet human needs.[24] In other words, patients, families, and staff concerns take priority over preparing for a meeting or justifying a budget variance.

At the beginning of each day, a "to do" list should be made in descending order of priority. Unanticipated problems may occur throughout the day, so priorities will need to be reset. This is common and really no different from when the manager was a staff nurse.

TIPS TO HELP DEAL WITH THE WORKLOAD

✔ Make a "to do" list.

✔ Organize your office by labeling file folders for each staff member, for staff meeting agenda items, and for issues to discuss with your supervisor.

✔ Place agendas and minutes of all meetings you attend in folders.

✔ Delegate activities to others when possible.

✔ Always question whether a problem or an issue is yours to own or whether it is better handled by another person.

✔ Organize communication with staff members by using bulletin boards and communication books.

✔ Always carry a calendar and write down standing meetings, lunch, and other appointments.

✔ Schedule time in your calendar for planning and organizing.

One trap new nurse managers fall into is that of trying to solve everything for everybody. In their eagerness to prove themselves to their subordinates, they take on the world. This does nothing more than frustrate the manager, if not immediately, then in time. Be very careful of reverse delegation by your staff. It is wise to adopt a coaching attitude, assisting them in solving the problem and implementing the solution, rather than ending up with all the problems heaped on your back. Solving problems can help the staff grow professionally as well as give them a different perspective.

Sooner or later the supervisor's priorities will clash with those of the manager. Rather than becoming frustrated, do not be afraid to negotiate a change in the project or the timeline.

SUMMARY

Knowledge of current NCDSs being practiced can help the new nurse manager in evaluating her own system. Knowledge of more recent concepts of restructured, patient-centered care, shared governance, and professional practice models is essential as the nurse manager leads her staff in providing quality, cost-effective care to patients and families.

Understanding and using a patient classification system, together with a master staffing plan for the area, assists the new nurse manager to staff the area efficiently and effectively. There are always concerns about liability connected with staffing.

Issues concerning credentialing are important to learn, especially the issue of continued competency of the nursing staff.

Mastering the ability to lead efficient and effective meetings is of high priority, as is that of facilitating clinical conferences.

Learning to prioritize duties, including time management, is a necessity for the nurse manager, whose work never seems to be done. Making rounds in the patient area assists in maintaining visibility as well as in accomplishing many other managerial tasks.

Finally, internalizing JCAHO standards helps the nurse manager in decision making, which helps her unit achieve and maintain quality nursing care.

REFERENCES

1. Manthey M: Structuring work around patients, *Nurs Manage* 20(5): 28, 1989.
2. Wake MM: Nursing care delivery systems: status and vision, *J Nurs Adm* 20(5):47, 1990.
3. Manthey M: Delivery systems and practice models: a dynamic balance, *Nurs Manage* 22(1):29, 1991.
4. American Hospital Association's Center for Nursing Survey: *1989 Hospital nursing personnel survey,* 1989, The AHA.
5. Sherman RO: Team nursing revisited, *J Nurs Adm* 20(11):44, 1990.
6. Munson FC, et al: *Nursing assignment patterns user's manual,* Ann Arbor, Mich, 1980, AUPHA Press.
7. Piltz-Kirkby M: The nursing assignment pattern study in practice, *Nurs Manage* 22(5):96HH, 1991.
8. Joint Commission on the Accreditation of Healthcare Organizations: *Accreditation manual for hospitals—volume I: standards,* Chicago, 1991, Joint Commission on the Accreditation of Healthcare Organizations.
9. Porter-O-Grady T: Shared governance for nursing, *AORN J* 53(2): 459, 1991.
10. Rose M, DiPasquale B: The Johns Hopkins professional practice model. In Mayer GG, Madden MJ, Lawrenz E, editors: *Patient care delivery models,* Rockville, Md, 1990, Aspen Publishers.
11. Lawrenz E, Mayer GG: Compensation for professional practice: an incentive model. In Mayer GG, Madden MJ, Lawrenz E, editors: *Patient care delivery models,* Rockville, Md, 1990, Aspen Publishers.
12. Perry L: Group practice model brings nursing unit's turnover to nil, *Mod Healthcare* 20:90, 1990.
13. Giovannetti P: *Patient classification for nurse staffing: criteria for selection and implementation,* Edmonton, Can-

ada, 1983, Alberta Association of Registered Nurses.

14. Nagaprasanna BR: Patient classification systems: strategies for the 1990s, *Nurs Manage* 19(3):105, 1988.

15. Barrett S: *Executive summary of 1990 National Nurse Manager Study by American Organization of Nurse Executives,* Chicago, 1991, American Hospital Association.

16. Huey FL, Hartley S: What keeps nurses in nursing—3,500 nurses tell their stories, *Am J Nurs* 88(2):181-188, 1988.

17. Ringl KK, Dotson L: Self scheduling for professional nurses, *Nurs Manage* 20(2):42, 1989.

18. Fiesta J: The nursing shortage: whose liability problem, Part II, *Nurs Manage* 21(2):22, 1990.

19. Fiesta J: Agency nurses—whose liability? *Nurs Manage* 21(3):16, 1990.

20. Baillie VK, Trygstad L, Cordoni TI: *Effective nursing leadership—a practical guide,* Rockville, Md, 1989, Aspen Publishers.

21. Lewis EM, Spicer JG: *Human resource management handbook—contemporary strategies for nursing managers,* Rockville, Md, 1987, Aspen Publishers.

22. Mahan F: Patient care conferences: a model, *Nurs Manage* 19(7):60, 1988.

23. Stevens BJ: *The nurse as executive,* ed 3, Rockville, Md, 1985, Aspen Publishers.

24. Seven ways to sharpen your leadership skills, *Nursing '89* 19(10):130, 1989.

Effective Time Management and Productivity

T. M. Marrelli

Effective time management is vital to accomplishing all work. Time management problems are easy to recognize; there is always too much pending work. The symptoms are papers piled high in baskets and stacks on your desk, notes attached to your office door, unread mail, and the inability to locate a specific piece of paper when you need it. The behavioral signs include thinking about the next project while discussing a current one, procrastinating about picking up the top piece of paper for fear of what's underneath, and forgetting appointments. These problems can be remedied. Effective time management, or habits that contribute to the effective use of this limited commodity, can be learned. More importantly, habits that are no longer efficient for you can be discarded. Working smarter, not harder, demands setting priorities, delegating effectively, and using other time management skills to achieve personal and organizational goals.

THE THREE *P*s OF PROCRASTINATION

Three *P*s may especially impede competent nurse managers from accomplishing dreaded work. These are:

1. Procrastination
2. Perfectionism
3. Prioritizing

Procrastination is generally defined as habitually postponing performance of burdensome tasks. Symptoms may include multiple stacks of paper on your desk overflowing onto credenzas, unopened mail, or the feeling of not wanting to go to work for fear of not meeting a deadline on a project. The problem with procrastination is that it is a learned habit. Like all habits, it can be unlearned and replaced with more successful behaviors. Examples of procrastination are delaying finalizing the minutes of the last product selection committee until the night before the next meeting or delaying performance evaluations because they are time-consuming. When this occurs, the added stress and pressure become greater than if the minutes had been completed earlier or if one performance evaluation was completed every afternoon. All of a sudden, routine items take on immense importance and a dread of not meeting deadlines sets in.

It is interesting to note that in Webster's New World Dictionary,[1] the word *deadline* has its origins as a "line around a prison beyond which a prisoner could go only at the risk of being shot." It is no wonder that we take deadlines seriously and feel impending discomfort as they approach and we are not or perceive we are not *ready*. This feeling usually lasts until the work is accomplished, then tremendous relief is felt. Also, while working, a realization usually is made—the task was not as bad as anticipated, or such a delay should not occur again because it takes too much energy. It is at this point that a conscious effort and decision must be made to change the habit of procrastination. Everyone endures certain job aspects that they do not enjoy. However, these dreaded duties grow in importance and cast a shadow on all other activities until completed. Just "doing it" results in incredible relief. In addition, it usually takes less time and energy than was anticipated. Most importantly, the feeling of accomplishment and satisfaction when done can reinforce the new just-do-it habit the next time. Therefore, when you initially get these dreaded uncomfortable feelings, it usually means you should do this job first and stop procrastinating.

Perfectionism is known generally to mean that work is never perceived to be "good enough." Perfectionists usually procrastinate because at some level they believe that no product is better than a poor product. Although this is not true, we all have known successful, competent people who function with these beliefs. If this sounds familiar, it is important to realize that, generally, any work product is better than none, and you may never have the luxury of time or other resources to accomplish a given project in the manner you believe it should be accomplished. Trying to be perfect wastes time and is an unrealistic goal. This is perhaps one of the most frustrating aspects of being a manager; not only will your work product often be incorporated into your supervisor's project, but in the end it may not resemble the same product at all. In management, you must make it okay (to yourself) for your managers to "own" parts of your work and recognize that you cannot control your product once it is submitted to your manager.

Prioritizing is the decision-making process that results in a systematic order in which to accomplish identified tasks. Prioritizing leads to organization, which is vital to effective time management.

Prioritizing can be closely linked to perfectionism and procrastination in two ways: (1) putting off or delaying what you do not want to do (procrastination) can result in those tasks being relegated to the end of your list of priorities, and (2) avoidance of starting and completing a task moves other tasks toward the end of the priority list. As the dread of deadline looms, there are seemingly endless lists of newer items given higher priority. It is at this point that the perfectionist starts believing that it's just too late for an acceptable product to even be created.

Though it is hard, *do* the most difficult task first. Even a draft of the project will give you some sense of accomplishment and a feeling of control over your work environment. The difficult tasks we put off are what become bigger and cause stress in the workplace. Doing the dreaded task will give you a sense of relief, rejuvenation, and accomplishment.

THE RIGHT STUFF ATTITUDES

Kenneth Pelletier of the University of California San Francisco School of Medicine conducted an ongoing study of executives in the telecommunications industry, as reported by Olsen.[2] The telecommunications industry has been plagued by turmoil and changes. It was found through this study that the people who thrived on the continual fast-paced changes shared some common beliefs. Some of these lessons may be applicable to the health care setting because of the dynamic and ever-changing environment health care managers face daily. The following tips for thriving on change may help you be an effective manager in today's fast-paced health care environment.

TIPS FOR THRIVING

✔ **Challenge**—Do not view change as a threat. Perceive it as a challenge and the chance or opportunity to do something new and innovative.

✔ **Control**—Believe that you can make an impact or a difference. This is probably the most important trait for thriving in a changing environment.

✔ **Commitment**—Get involved and active in the new ideas and change. Do not deny the reality of the changing situation.

✔ **Social support**—Use your friends, family, and colleagues for support. It helps to have a sense of working and pulling together. Your network does not have to be large, just established and used. Pelletier says, "It's enough that you have a supportive, trusting relationship with the person at the next desk."[2] (This reinforces the importance and need for peer support among nurse managers.)

✔ **Stress management**—Learn your own stress signals. Pelletier found that the healthiest executives all knew what to do when their stress levels got too high. He said methods for relief varied and the one chosen did not matter. For this group, methods included listening to music and various other methods that worked. Relieving stress is vital to reenergizing oneself.[2]

If you believe that you are alone in struggling to effectively manage your time, consider this thought. Large[3] states, "More new information has been produced in the last 30 years than in the previous 5,000 . . . and the total of all printed knowledge doubles every 8 years." There is clearly too much information and not enough time to incorporate it. What is more, not all information received is pertinent or relevant to the task at hand. The new term that has been created for this overwhelming amount of knowledge is *information anxiety.* In addition to this overload, you may have sales representatives and other vendors who wish to further increase your knowledge of the particular product or service they are selling. Finally, your life does not comprise only work (though in difficult times it can certainly *feel* that way), and you may receive additional information daily through your personal mail and phone.

The good news is anyone can become organized. Contrary to belief, your desk does not need to be neat and clean to be organized. Tidiness works for some, whereas others can locate any needed piece of paper on what appears to be a messy desk. You can be more organized and use your limited time more effectively. The skills and time management tips recommended in this chapter can also be extended into your home.

THREE WAYS TO HANDLE PAPER

✔ Act on it

✔ File it

✔ Discard it

✔ Regardless of the chosen category, try to handle it only once.

Handling Paper

Act-on-it items include action items such as memos needing response, confirmation of meeting attendance, scheduling changes, and other situations where your immediate input is needed.

Discard-it items include advertisements for various services or products that are not appropriate for your area and memos sent to you as occupant nurse manager or confirmation memos that need no further action on your part.

File-it items include items that may need retrieval in the future (e.g., communications from your manager, HR issues, and other important documentation).

The main difficulty in this process is deciding what to file and what to discard. You can learn a lot about the nurse manager who preceded you and the filing system that may be acceptable at your work setting by reviewing the remaining files. The core files may include HR files, copies of patient complaints that may or may not have been forwarded to the patient omsbudman and/or risk manager, clinical and management articles circulated to all managers from administration, and voluminous paper communications sent to or from the unit.

You do not have to keep every piece of paper to be an effective nurse manager. Ask your peers what information they keep and what they discard. Avoid the tendency to be a pack rat.

23 TIPS TO HELP YOU MANAGE TIME

✔ Recognize that time is a scarce and nonrenewable resource.

✔ Remember that being organized is a key component of effective time management.

✔ Evaluate your own use of time. Keep a log for 2 weeks and note the activities and time allotted for them. Keep another log after implementing these suggestions to see if measurable improvements in your work output occur.

✔ Understand that everyone has her own organization style. You do not have to have a neat and spotless desk to be organized. Some very organized managers have messy desks but can put their hands on any piece of paper when needed.

✔ Know that successful, busy people usually have effective personal organizational skills.

✔ Schedule time to file or do paperwork *every* day. Start files for such ongoing business as leave requests, unit activity reports, or QA/QI minutes.

✔ Prioritize tasks on a daily basis.

✔ Schedule and meet deadlines.

✔ Formulate realistic goals and break them down into tasks by creating short-range goals. When all these tasks are completed, long-term objectives will have been achieved. Break down all large jobs into small pieces. Schedule time to do the small pieces.

✔ Maintain your flexibility. Reorder priorities whenever indicated based on organizational needs.

✔ Know that if something is not a priority or important, it may not need to be done.

✔ Visualize yourself learning to effectively cope with change, turmoil, and chaos. With this attitude, it will not unduly upset you when it happens.

✔ Managing your own time effectively will result in more efficient use of staff time as your actions are copied.

✔ Accept that your schedule may change based on many situations, such as your manager's needs, a clinical problem, or an unscheduled lengthy disaster drill on your unit.

✔ Maximize your use of time because this improves overall performance and contributes to cost containment goals.

✔ Know that planning and delegation are vital to organizational and personal goal achievement.

✔ Realize that an effective time manager gets more accomplished, has improved quality of work, meets deadlines and other commitments, and increases effectiveness overall.

✔ Make and use "to do" lists or planners whenever possible.

✔ Take the last few minutes of your work day to reflect on your accomplishments and to prioritize the tasks of the next day. Feel satisfied with those completed tasks and the job you are doing.

✔ You can have an open-door policy and attitude without the door always literally being open. Staff should have access, but you can control that access.

✔ Pick a regularly scheduled day, (e.g., every third Tuesday) for clearing off your desk totally and reprioritizing big projects.

✔ Use the phone whenever possible—it may save you writing a memo and time-consuming communications.

✔ Check off tasks as completed—it feels great!

30 ACTION TIPS TO HELP YOU MANAGE YOUR ENVIRONMENT

✔ Hang a large calendar in an accessible area on which you and your staff can identify vacations, in-services, or scheduled absences. If feasible, it is particularly helpful if you are able to read this at a glance from your desk phone.

✔ Choose the style of "to do" list that works best for you. Try different ones until you decide which method suits you best.

✔ Identify your peak work time. Try to schedule the most intense or important tasks during this time.

✔ Concentrate on the task at hand by controlling distractions. It is okay to schedule time for you; close your office door.

✔ Leave the work area, when possible, for at least a few minutes a day. Take a lunch or other meal break, even if it means just shutting your door and eating an apple in peace.

✔ Place mailboxes for your staff in an easily accessible place for your use. Mailboxes can be used for scheduling, feedback, and delegated work.

✔ Schedule time for all routine duties; otherwise they probably will not get done. For example, schedule time to review performance evaluations and other on-going unit activity tasks. If it is not scheduled, it is not respected as a priority.

✔ Learn to use a computer for all written products. The editing, spelling checkers, and thesaurus tools are an immense help when memos or reports are due. When you use a computer, organize your disks in a manner effective for you. Remember to keep the phone, scissors, or other magnetic material away from your computer and the disks because such items may erase hours of hard work.

✔ Practice speedreading or proofreading skills if your position uses those special skills.

✔ Organize your phone numbers in a systematic way. This method should be whatever works and is easiest for you. Have the most frequently called numbers accessible and placed near your phone.

✔ Control interruptions for certain periods of each day. The ability to do this effectively will vary based on the work setting and other factors.

✔ Refer to a thesaurus and a recent edition dictionary located on your desk whenever creating written products.

✔ Maintain and update a desk calendar or other organizer to determine your planned daily, weekly, and monthly schedules.

✔ Create an office environment that promotes work completion while also reflecting your personality.

✔ Organize and update your business phone numbers and addresses on a regularly scheduled basis.

✔ Make your environment work for you. Sometimes it may be appropriate to go the hospital library to research a project for presentation. Other times, just closing your office door may be sufficient.

✔ Remember that becoming and staying organized is a learned skill and that, with practice, good habits can replace bad ones.

✔ Believe that you can not do everything for everyone else and still achieve your goals.

✔ Use your interpersonal skills to politely end conversations. When phoning people known to be long-winded, set up the conversation to be short. This can be achieved in a couple of ways: (1) "Dr. No, this is Nurse Manager, I have only a minute between meetings to return your call and tell you. . . .," or (2) "Well, I've got to go, I think my manager is on the other line" or "I have a call I've been expecting and have to go." Your pager can also be used for this purpose.

✔ Practice visualization daily, seeing yourself as a calm and effective manager.

✔ Begin every morning by taking 3 minutes to relax and focus on the day's tasks ahead. With practice, this exercise will keep you centered throughout the day on your priorities.

✔ Listen to *any* recommendations that have the possibility of being a more efficient and successful way of doing things. Stop yourself the moment your automatic response begins with, "But it's always been done this way." That alone is usually a good reason to revaluate the way something is done.

✔ Learn to say "no" and mean it.

✔ Be flexible in the time parameters set in your schedule. If you overschedule your time and consistently run over, you will feel even more harried and hassled. Allot sufficient time between scheduled activities.

✔ Accept that there will *always* be interruptions. This is part of being a manager. The key is controlling and balancing them. Evaluate your office space: is the furniture in a configuration that is conducive to decreasing or minimizing interruptions?

✔ Teach your staff that whenever a problem is brought to your attention, you will hear it only if a recommended solution is attached.

✔ Visualize yourself as an innovative, creative thinker and problem solver.

✔ Practice relaxation techniques and deep breathing exercises on a regular basis.

✔ Take breaks. These are very important. Take them, do not feel guilty, and savor them. The restorative power of a break leaves you with more energy while increasing your productivity.

✔ Take great care of yourself. Get a massage, have manicures, exercise, eat well, play golf, or whatever *you like to do*. Effective time management will allow more time for those activities.

THE IMPORTANCE OF DELEGATION

It has been said that the effective use of time, or time management, is more about management than about time. With this in mind, you will find that your staff is vital to accomplishing all work. Delegation is the tool that transfers the work to your subordinates. Delegation gives the nursing staff responsibility, which contributes to a sense of belonging and accomplishment. Successful completion of the duties delegated empowers and develops the staff member to whom the work was delegated. In decentralized organizations, delegation is key to work accomplishment. The nurse manager must achieve organizational and unit goals, and the ordering of the priorities and the management of the time allotted in which to do them is of great importance. The more responsibilities a person assumes and the busier a person becomes, the more effective delegation becomes the essential tool to accomplish work and achieve goals.

14 TIPS TO DELEGATE EFFECTIVELY

✔ Believe it is *not* easier or quicker to do it yourself. (It is not!)

✔ Realize you must delegate to accomplish work.

✔ Learn to delegate wherever possible; it frees you up to manage and it develops your staff.

✔ Delegate by stating clearly the work and the product expected; specify deadlines, including a date on which you want a draft or the product; state that you be apprised of progress weekly and that you want immediate notification if a problem is impeding completion by the due date.

✔ Give feedback, positive wherever possible, on the progress and on the final product. Share comments from others on the work product where possible. For example, if your manager compliments the work and writes you a note about it, share the note with the staff member who created the product. It also is helpful to keep such notes in the staff member's personnel file on the unit so that during performance evaluation, you remember work products accomplished and the feedback received.

✔ Teach and direct your staff to use each other as resources. This creates an atmosphere of autonomy and professionalism that keeps nurses satisfied with their jobs.

✔ Delegate initially to those who are assertive or have told you that they want more responsibility. At first it may be truly difficult to delegate; but give this attitude up. Believe that your staff will do a good job. Resist the temptation to meddle in delegated projects.

✔ Expect the best from your staff and chances are you will get it.

✔ Remember that working in an environment where autonomy and independence are valued is considered an asset by nurses and assists in nurse retention. Make that the environment where you are the nurse manager.

✔ Staff members should know they can make mistakes and recommend solutions and improvements.

✔ Be professional. Do not denigrate your staff or their work to anyone; it comes back around and does not support an environment conducive to effective team-building.

✔ Remember the concepts of accountability, responsibility, and authority when delegating. Work may not be done the same way you would have done it, but it was completed and you did not have to do it personally.

✔ Offer a choice in the duties needing delegation when possible. This encourages staff growth and autonomy.

✔ Realize what should not be delegated. This may include HR issues, any confidential issues, delicate political problems with other departments or units, conflicts started by "he said/she said" scenarios, and complaints/communications with physicians or visitors that have risk management implications.

RESOURCES FOR TIME MANAGEMENT

There are ways to improve time management. It is important to be open to new ideas. The resources discussed below are those which should be considered where possible.

Using Computers in Nursing

The time management implications of information systems for nurses and nurse managers is currently being discussed in all health settings and in the literature. Automation in documentation should be fully explored because documentation continues to be an area of duplicative actions and inefficient use of the professional nurse's limited time. Computers are encouraging a shift toward standardized care plans and other automated data trends. This needs to occur given the following information. The American Hospital Association[4] (AHA) says that patient charts now average 70 to 100 pages. Medical records departments in most mid-sized hospitals process some 250,000 to 360,000 pieces of information each year. Because a patient's medical record may be reviewed as many as 30 times and stored for up to 30 years, more than 90% of hospitals have turned to computers to manage the information.

Computerized nursing documentation is becoming more common in health settings as applications for automation in nursing have increased. In some systems, the nurse can identify those actions or findings appropriate to a specific patient to facilitate the clinical entry. Computerization, particularly at the patient's bedside, assists in ensuring frequent, timely nursing entries. Computerizing the record and the nursing notes and other entries may ultimately save hospitals money and increase the quality of care provided. Studies have shown that nursing costs can account for 30% to 40% of a hospital's operational budget. It has been estimated that 2 to 3 hours of a nursing shift is spent performing administrate tasks.[5] Nursing computer systems available today are integrating the different components of the chart. For example, once the assessment is completed, an individualized care plan is developed. From that point, a patient-specific flow chart can be generated, thus decreasing the documentation process by 40% to 50% per nurse per shift. Kardexes and other pieces of information can also be developed via a computer system. Computerizing nursing documentation may be the next step in decreasing repetitive and duplicative administrative tasks. The confidentiality issues of computerized entries and retrieval of needed information are important factors currently being addressed by both systems users and developers. The growing specialty of nursing informatics is one resource available to nurse managers that facilitates the move toward automation in the work setting.

Detail Management (or, When You Cannot See the Forest for the Trees)

Undoubtedly, it is easy to be overwhelmed and burdened with details. Minutia can leave you exhausted before you even begin your first priority task. Details that belong to a bigger project should be written down and placed in the folder for that project. Other details should be judged as to whether they have true value or can be thrown away.

Delegate the resolution of some of these details back to the staff members who brought them to you. As with all duties delegated, give a deadline for when you want a report on the outcome. An example could be the completion of meeting minutes that both you and a staff member attended. The staff member can use both your notes to effectively complete the assignment.

The Value of Unit Activity Reports

The monthly or quarterly operational or unit reports can be an effective tool for demonstrating work that has been accomplished in the clinical area in a specific time frame. They are also effective tools for evaluation, reassessing how work is done on your unit, or justifying additional resources. Although these reports can be perceived as one more administrative chore, they are quantifiable and objective information about the work achieved with you as nurse manager. The format may change at varied health settings, but it generally includes such concise information as the following:

1. Actual (to date) versus projected (budgeted) expenses
2. An update on QA/QI activities
3. Personnel/staffing update, including staffing patterns and full-time equivalent (FTE) vacancies
4. In-service programs or other educational programs held
5. Average patient length of stay (LOS) and occupancy rates
6. Any major accomplishments or unusual problems
7. Update on the unit's activities in areas such as practice or research committees
8. Number of visits or patient encounters completed
9. Other data specific to your area (e.g., incident reports)

These reports can also be a valuable source of information for the nurse manager's performance evaluation. It will assist in remembering special projects or unusual episodes on your unit. These reports can also bring a feeling of accomplishment when there is no perception of closure because of ongoing problems and processes on the unit. When this is the case, these reports can give the professional nurse manager a sense of accomplishment and a job well done.

SUMMARY

Effective time management results in quality work produced by set deadlines. It also develops staff initiative and personal growth through effective use of delegation by the nurse manager. The nurse manager who practices effective time management skills acts as a role model to both staff and peers. It has been said that, "Misuse of time seldom involves an isolated incident. It is usually part of a well-established pattern of behavior." These patterns of behavior, or habits, can be changed.[6]

Greater job satisfaction is achieved through work being accomplished; all work entails time management skills. The improvement of these key skills will increase productivity on the unit, which in turn reinforces sound habits of time management. The nurse manager sees increased quality of care and improved morale in an atmosphere that fosters staff growth and autonomy. Time management is vital to the successful operation of any health care setting and to the personal health and professional growth of a nurse manager.

REFERENCES

1. *Webster's New World Dictionary of the American Language,* second college ed, New York, 1982, Simon and Schuster.
2. Olsen E: Beyond positive thinking, *J Nurs Adm* 20(5):11, 1990.
3. Large P: *The micro revolution revisited,* Totowa, NJ, 1984, Rowman & Allenheld.
4. American Hospital Association: *Side-by-side profiles,* Medical records: increasing importance, heavier workload, pp 1-4, Chicago, 1990, The AHA.
5. Carter K: Computer technology advances will help hospitals to compete, *Modern Healthcare* 15(24):90-92, 1985.
6. Bliss EC: *Getting things done,* NY, 1976, Bantam Books.

CHAPTER 7

Budgeting Basics

Lynda Hilliard

Total quality management (TQM), continuous quality improvement (CQI), consumer awareness of health care issues, limited health care resources, and an increasing need for more health care services to an aging and AIDS-infected society are revolutionizing health care. Not only is the nurse manager responsible for providing high-quality patient care, but also for achieving that goal with fiscally sound, effective methods.

The days of cost-based reimbursement for hospital care are past. High-quality, goal-oriented, predictable, and affordable health care is demanded by all segments of society and has become the focus of recent state and presidential political campaigns. Hospitals and their managers must be able to provide that type of service to survive in America's demanding health care marketplace.

TOTAL QUALITY MANAGEMENT

TQM principles have been derived from the business sector and applied to health care objectives. Competition, scarce economic resources, and societal demand for quality care at a reasonable price are all factors forcing hospital administrators to conserve limited resources by streamlining operations while continuing to provide "user-friendly" service to their customers. TQM is a process that not only focuses on fixing problems, but that also continually searches for methods to improve and make more cost-effective the delivery of services.[1]

TQM has provided the impetus for staff members from all segments of a hospital environment to meet, prioritize goals, and cross traditional career boundaries to develop and test methods to better serve their customers. Examples of quality action teams (QATs) that have addressed challenging hospital-based issues at a small, urban California hospital include the following:

- Outpatient department wait times
- Back safety/productivity costs
- Patient transport issues
- Medication errors

All of the above QATs had staff members from various departments investigate and research the relevant issues and leave their territorial concerns behind as they searched for solutions that would enhance and improve the delivery of patient care. Patient satisfaction will ultimately be achieved. Also, this continuous review of operations will eventually make the organization more cost-effective—a needed ingredient in the health care arena of the 1990s. For a more detailed view of TQM, please refer to Chapter 9.

DIAGNOSTIC-RELATED GROUPS

Managers must understand the types and complexities of the resources needed to achieve patient care goals, and they also must be aware of the fiscal constraints placed on operations for the proper use of limited resources.

Diagnostic-related groups (DRGs) is a classification system that was developed in the 1980s and adapted by the Health Care Financing Administration (HCFA) to control the cost of health care to its Medicare beneficiaries.

Before the advent of DRGs, most nurse managers were not actively involved in the budget process. However, nurse managers are now responsible for the development of their unit's budget and maintaining cost of operations within the stated budget at most health care institutions.

Positive performance evaluations and career progression within the health care setting depend on a manager's fiscal knowledge and responsibility, as well as clinical expertise.

COST-BASED REIMBURSEMENT

After the advent of the Medicare program in 1967 and before the 1980s, hospitals were reimbursed on a cost basis. Basically, cost-based reimbursement for the Medicare program classified the various costs of operating a hospital, noted the number of patients served, determined the average cost per patient, and then reimbursed the hospital for all Medicare patients.

Through this generous but inefficient system, hospitals were able to expand at a record pace and provide a wide array of very expensive, often duplicative, services without any incentive to economize. All costs were passed on to the consumer through the third-party payer (insurance companies, state Medicaid programs, and especially the federal government through the Medicare program). Health care costs rose much faster than did the rate of inflation during the years following the inception of the Medicare program.

Today, nurse executives, chief executive officers, chief operations officers, and chief financial officers daily review and analyze the financial operations of their institutions. Operational decisions are made quickly to react to adverse conditions (e.g., negative payer mix, low census, or rising staffing costs not related to increased volumes) that may endanger the financial situation of a hospital or agency.

The nurse manager must continually view the nursing unit in the same way—as a viable business. Managers must be able to react to financial changes immediately. To do that, the effective nurse manager must understand the complexities and terminology of the fiscal process to be able to react quickly to change. At the end of this chapter, a glossary of financial terms is available for review.

FISCAL MANAGEMENT

The senior managerial staff is responsible to the governing body or board of directors of the hospital or agency for the effective management of that institution. The proper management of a hospital's or agency's finances is just as important as is the provision of quality patient care services. A hospital or other health program cannot survive in the 1990s without a fiscally astute management team. To understand fiscal management, a few basic concepts must be learned.

Fiscal or financial management is derived from basic accounting principles. According to Shillinglaw and Meyer,[2] "Accounting is the primary financial method of gathering, organizing and presenting information that can be utilized by management and outsiders in evaluating an organization."

As with all professional disciplines, accounting uses methods or measurements that follow prescribed rules to provide standardized analysis when comparing one institution with another.[3]

Hospitals and other health care organizations follow the standards of the JCAHO to prove the quality of their services. Accounting practices are governed by the Financial Accounting Standards Board, which issues statements of financial accounting standards.

DEFINITION OF ASSETS, LIABILITIES, AND NET WORTH

The most fundamental accounting maxim is:

Assets = Liabilities + Owner's equity (net worth)

✔ An **asset** is any property (tangible or intangible) that is owned by the institution (e.g., cash, accounts receivable, and property).

✔ A **liability** is a debt that the institution owes to other businesses and/or individuals, such as accounts payable and mortgages.

✔ **Net worth,** or **owner's equity,** constitutes worth in terms of monies that would be divided among the owners if the institution were to go out of business.

NONPROFIT VERSUS PROFIT STATUS

In the health care arena, hospitals are generally nonprofit institutions, making them tax-exempt. In years of efficient operations, hospitals list their excess revenues over expenses as a positive fund balance, or net worth.

In a for-profit business, a positive fund balance would be called profit and divided among stockholders in the form of a dividend, or it would be reinvested in the business. In a nonprofit hospital, excess monies should thus be reinvested in the facility and/or in expanding services provided to the community it serves.

CAPITAL EXPANSION OR REINVESTMENT

Prudent business managers realize the need for a business to reinvest in its plant and facilities to maintain viable operations. Generally, health care institutions must realize an annual net gain of at least 5% (based on revenues over expenses) to replace assets as needed.

Many hospitals have historically derived a percentage of income from sources other than operations (e.g., fund-raising and interest or dividends on investments). However, this is not a sound practice. The hospital budget should reflect expenses that can be covered by anticipated revenues from operations. It should not count on investment income to cover general expenses of daily operations. The situation is comparable to a family living beyond the earnings of the breadwinners and tapping savings accounts or investment accounts on a consistent basis. In such a case, annual family budgets are developed and include savings account income to cover expenses. After a short time, that source of income is depleted and the family has lost in two ways: (1) those emergency monies or special-project monies are gone, and (2) the family has built a lifestyle that the annual salary of the breadwinners cannot support.

PUBLIC PERCEPTION OF HOSPITALS

During the past few years, national controversy has risen in the health care community regarding the public perception of hospitals being managed as businesses. Recent tax rulings by the Internal Revenue Service have pitted revenue-starved communities against major hospitals and/or medical centers. At stake are large amounts of property tax revenues being waived because of the nonprofit status of health care institutions. The tax-exempt status of such "profitable" institutions, which are perceived as either limiting access or refusing health care to those community members without insurance and/or the financial resources to pay for their care, is under review.

The historical public view of hospitals as being charitable institutions providing care for all who come to their doors is being transformed into the view of a large, multifaceted corporation whose primary mission is to produce a positive bottom line, as evidenced by intense competition for paying patients. In the future, more institutions will be challenged about their tax-exempt status as local governing agencies examine the financial activities of their community-based hospital against its mission statement.

The successful hospital management team will plan with their governing body to effectively recognize and integrate the health care needs of their community into their strategic plan, while conserving resources and maintaining a positive bottom line.

FINANCIAL PERFORMANCE REPORTS

The formal reports that measure a hospital's financial performance are the *financial statements,* which include the income and expense statement and the balance sheet.

Income and Expense Statement

The income and expense statement lists all the revenues, expenses, and net income or (loss) for a given period, usually on a monthly or annual basis. Any type of revenue can constitute income (e.g., dividends or interest on investments). In a business, the entity should operate on the income generated from the service it provides. See Figure 7-1 for a sample income and expense statement.

Balance Sheet

The balance sheet lists an institution's assets, liabilities, and net worth, as of a specific date. All an organization's assets must equal the total of the liabilities and net worth (fund balance) combined. To be in balance, the two totals must equal. Figure 7-2 is an example of a balance sheet.

Seaside Hospital
Operating Income and Expense Statement
January 1—December 31, 1991
($000)

Gross revenues		$76,000
Deductions	$(25,000)	
Net revenue		$51,000
Operating expenses		
Salary costs	$25,000	
Other	15,000	
Bond expense	4,000	(44,000)
Net Income		$ 7,000

FIG. 7-1   An income and expense statement.

Seaside Hospital
Balance Sheet
December 31, 1991
($000)

ASSETS
Current assets:

Cash		$ 2
Accounts receivable*		6
Inventories		2
Total current assets		$10
Land, plant, and equipment	$20	
Less: accum depreciation	8	12
Total Assets		$22

LIABILITIES AND NET WORTH
Current liabilities

Accounts payable†	$ 4
Notes payable	1
Total current liabilities	$ 5
Bonds payable	3
Total liabilities	$ 8

Net worth

Retained earnings	$14
Total Liabilities and Net Worth	$22

*Accounts receivable is classified as asset becuase it is the amount of money owed to the hospital for the services already rendered (i.e., insurances billed, but money not yet received).

†Accounts payable is classified a liability because it is a cumulation of all the debts owed vendors for services already rendered to the hospital that will be paid for within the year.

FIG. 7-2   A balance sheet.

INSURANCE OVERVIEW

As stated earlier, hospitals are generally paid for their services by third-party payers, as opposed to individual payers or self-pay. The process of indirect payment from individuals for their care has been part of the national debate over the rising costs of health care. In the past, consumers never felt the pinch of high health care costs because their insurance companies paid the bill and their employers paid the cost of the insurance premium. However, recently, as insurance companies raise their premiums drastically to meet rising costs and employers are unable to meet the increased payments, the consumer has been forced to bear a larger portion (deductible) of the costs, thereby becoming acutely aware of the high cost of health care and the need to conserve and use services sparingly and appropriately.

In this section, different methods of insurance coverage are briefly described. Insurance coverage packages are ever-evolving, as providers of health care services develop mechanisms to attract the health care dollar and/or insurance premium.

Types of Insurance Plans

Indemnity

Indemnity insurance is a health care insurance plan that provides a specified amount of money to the insured when certain events occur, but it does not guarantee complete coverage for the cost of the medical services.

Fee-for-Service Benefit Plan

Fee-for-service benefits are included in insurance plans that have generally paid for hospital services on a full-charge basis. Historically, these plans have imposed few, if any, limitations on health care providers (hospitals or physicians). Reimbursement has been based on three factors, as follows:

1. Indemnity fee schedules/predetermined payments per procedure or service
2. Usual, customary, and reasonable fee schedule
3. Relative value units, or the assignment of dollar values to a coded listing of services based on complexity of service

The two major categories of fee-for-service plans are as follows:

1. Basic hospitalization (with or without basic medical/surgical coverage)
2. Comprehensive hospitalization and medical/surgical coverage

Deductibles are usually associated with fee-for-service insurance arrangements; they are the amount of medical expenses that the individual must pay before a third-party payer will assume any liability for payment of benefits. The deductible can be either a fixed amount of money or the value of certain services over a given period (e.g., the deductible is equal to the charges for the first day of hospitalization).

As health care costs rose and insurance premiums followed, alternative delivery systems were developed to provide hospital and/or professional services on other than the charge, or fee-for-service, basis. Examples of alternative delivery systems include:

- Exclusive Provider Arrangement
- Health Maintenance Organization (HMO)
- Preferred Provider Organization (PPO)
- Individual Provider Arrangement (IPA)

Exclusive Provider Arrangement

An exclusive provider arrangement is a service plan that pays for health care services only if provided by contracted professional and/or institutional providers. This does not include emergency services or services required while out of the geographic service area.

Health Maintenance Organization

An HMO is a health care organization that provides comprehensive health services to its enrolled population for a fixed periodic payment.

Capitation is the term used to describe the fixed rate of payment (per member, per month) received by a health care provider on a periodic basis to cover a specified amount of health care services. All HMOs use a capitation rate when budgeting for their service area.

The ability to predict health plan premiums or costs based on the statistical analyses of financial, utilization, and demographic trends in a given area is found in actuarial services.

Preferred Provider Organization

A PPO is an organization of health care providers who have negotiated a special, usually reduced rate to attract insurance plan beneficiaries.

Individual Provider Arrangement

An IPA is an organization that contracts with health care providers for the provision of medical services in their own offices for prepaid or managed care plans. One of the first alternative delivery plans was the prepaid plan. This is an insurance plan that offers its enrollees a defined set of benefits provided by a panel of providers within a specified geographic area. Kaiser Permanente was one of the first employers on the West Coast that provided such a plan, starting about 50 years ago.

DISCOUNTED SERVICES

All of the above plans have common denominators, but the most striking for hospitals is that the plans demand discounted services. Discounts or deductions from revenue are the contracted amounts deducted from patient care revenues that the hospital must write off. Any or all of the alternative delivery plans may also negotiate a daily rate for the delivery of all hospital services or only selected services, regardless of the actual services provided.

For example, a hospital may have a discount arrangement with a local HMO stating that the HMO pays 80% of charges for guarantee of all local enrollees to be hospitalized at the contract hospital. The 20% difference would be deducted from the gross revenue, as well as the actual expense of providing the services. In most states, third-party payors are actively negotiating preferential rates with health care providers to try and control health care costs to their beneficiaries.

It is very important for all managers and their staff to understand the concept of discounted services. Many states have a multitude of insurance providers demanding discounted services before sending their enrollees to that facility. An example is a small California hospital that has at least 30 different contracts. Each plan may have different preauthorization rules, lengths of stay, and/or types of service requirements that must be observed, understood, and applied appropriately to maintain financial viability.

PAYOR MIX

A typical example of a payor mix at a small urban hospital in the San Francisco-Sacramento area is as follows:

49% Medicare
17% MediCal (Medicaid)
10% Commercial (100% of total charges paid)
19% HMO/PPO (discounted contracts)
5% Self-pay

As you can see, 85% of anticipated revenues have been or will be discounted—Medicare through the prospective payment system for DRGs; MediCal with a structured rate system; HMO/PPO through discounted arrangements; and, most probably, write offs for the self-pay (usually working individuals without insurance who do not qualify for Medicaid funds).

When charges are revised reflecting the increased cost of providing a service, the average discount is added back in to reflect true costs. In this scenario it is easy to comprehend why charges are rising so fast—to react to the demands for increased discounts from the payors. Staff members and managers need to understand the correlation between the gross charge and the net charge. In some cases, hospitals are averaging $.50 on the $1 of health care revenues because of discount arrangements.

CASE MANAGEMENT

Case management is the coordination of high-cost health care services provided to a patient according to specific diagnoses. Coordination of care is the primary goal of health care insurance providers. It should also be the goal of all health care providers.

At this time, health care delivery is disjointed. A patient may see three different physicians (specialists), each treating a different problem with different goals in mind.

Insurance carriers may use the services of a case management or utilization review organization. These companies have rapidly grown since 1988 to provide a unique service; they monitor the delivery of care to insurance enrollees and are, in effect, "gatekeepers" to providers of care.

Hospitals have had utilization review and case management specialists on staff for many years, usually RNs or medical social workers. Their goal is to review all patient medical records daily to make sure over-utilization of services is not occurring.

In the past few years, the roles of such professionals have expanded greatly to include monitoring patients with the provisions of their insurance plans in mind to ensure the facility will be reimbursed for the services rendered. They coordinate with the attending physician and the nursing staff to ensure the patient receives appropriate levels of care and that all insurance requirements for payment are met.

Many physicians openly resent or are leery of hospital-based or insurance carrier utilization review staffs, who they feel sit in judgement of their clinical practice and try to control or manipulate the amount or type of health care.

Studies and on-site clinical trials are occurring in various hospitals across the United States, developing and fine-tuning case management skills. Clinical pathways have been instituted that follow a diagnosis and/or surgical procedure and actually outline the types of services and levels of care required for that diagnosis. Barring complications, it also outlines what type and when the delivery of ancillary services, such as x-ray studies, will be allowed.

Clinical pathways use outcome criteria as an indicator of quality. The pathways require close cooperation between all health care providers in an institution to reach the expected outcome in the most efficient manner. In that way, TQM methods will greatly enhance the introduction of more case management models into hospitals in the future.

THE BUDGET PROCESS

A budget is a document that outlines, for a specific period (usually 1 year), the plan an organization has developed for the consumption of resources. It involves the forecasting of revenue-generating activities and the resources used to achieve those goals. Nurse managers are usually involved in the development of three types of budgets, as follows:

1. Capital
2. Operating
3. Personnel

There are also different types of budgets, varying according to how they are generated and viewed during the budget cycle. A budget cycle is the period of time that the budget addresses—monthly, yearly or multiple years. However, in most health care institutions, the budget cycle is on an annual basis following the fiscal year of the institution.

BUDGETING STYLES

✔ A **fixed budget** is a budget amount that does not fluctuate with volume or staffing levels.

✔ **A flexible budget** is a budget that can be adjusted either up or down depending on the volume of service, which gives a manager a more accurate accounting of the costs incurred during a certain time frame.

✔ **Zero-based budgeting** refers to the process of planning and reviewing operations from the bottom up. It is not just an add-on of a certain percentage each year to account for volume increases or other indicators. The manager must review the expected service, what resources that service will require, and the cost of each of the resources for inclusion on the requested budget.

Capital Budget

A capital budget outlines the forecasted buying of large, fixed assets or types of equipment that depreciate (e.g., furniture, buildings, diagnostic imaging equipment). Usually the finance department will generate a pay-back analysis before approving the purchase of such budget items to ascertain whether the equipment can generate enough revenue to pay itself off over a given amount of time.

Depreciation is the amount/portion or cost of an asset that can be attributed to a certain operating period. In other words, if an IV pump costs $500 and has a estimated life of 5 years, then the depreciation expense will be $100 per year and can be costed to the unit or area.

To meet government regulations, hospital capital budgets are forecasted over a 3-year period. However, they are reviewed and revised annually and as necessary as needs change. Figure 7-3 provides a sample capital acquisition summary.

Most payback analysis and net present value determinations can be generated with finance computer software. However, the nurse manager must supply the number of procedures and so forth that are estimated from the new piece of equipment, the amount of patient charge per procedure, and the total expense of operating the equipment. In that way, the finance department can determine whether the equipment can pay for itself within a stated period.

Seaside Hospital
Budget Calendar Year 1991
Captital Acquisition Summary
($500.00 or more per item and 3 or more years of useful life)

Dept prior	Proposed buy date	Item description	Replace/ upgrade	Number needed	Estimated cost of each	Estimated total cost (including tax)

Attach as much supporting data as possible for each item, along with Capital Budget Form C-1. Return to line administrator for review and approval by September 1, 1990.

_____ Department
Manager Signature   Date

_____ Line
Administrator Approval   Date

FIG. 7-3   A capital acquisition summary.

Not all capital expenditures should be analyzed on payback analysis and/or net present value. If equipment is needed for regulatory or safety reasons, those reasons should be documented first. However, the above method is a good way to determine the allocation of limited capital monies.

Operating Budget

An operating budget describes the day-to-day operational expenses of a unit (excluding personnel costs). These types of costs include, but are not limited to, medical and nonmedical supplies, electricity, small equipment items (usually under $300 to $500 [i.e., stethoscope or sphygmomanometer]), and outside education expenses.

Ideally, all unit managers should create budgets using the zero-based method. However, that is not always possible for all budget categories. For this reason, it is important for the new nurse manager to review all the budget categories used for the past few years and determine appropriateness and continued applicability.

The categories which can be determined as direct costs and to which zero-based budgeting can be applied make the forecast more realistic and sustainable. An example would be the budgeting for an oncology unit with an estimated 100 admissions over the next 12 months. If the standard protocol called for IV lines for each patient and the lines were to be changed every 24 hours, and the length of stay was averaged at 3 days per patient, the manager could get an approximation of how many tubing lines to order.

$$100 \text{ patients} \times 3 \text{ lines per patient} = 300 \text{ tubing lines}$$
$$300 \text{ lines} \times \$25 \text{ each} = \$750$$

Zero-based budgeting is very tedious, especially for a unit that uses a tremendous amount of supplies and/or other budgeted items. However, depending on the amount of time allotted to formulating budgets and the ability to control costs, it should be done at least every few years to determine accuracy and serve as a monitoring system.

Understanding how a cost has been applied to a budget and how the cost can be reduced from a budget allows the nurse manager more fiscal control of the unit. It also makes reporting and understanding variances much easier to learn.

Personnel Budget

Finally, a personnel or full-time equivalent (FTE) budget is the document that forecasts the actual need for unit staff 24 hours per day, 365 days per year. Nursing personnel or FTE budgets differ from those of other hospital departments in that, in addition to the estimated number of patient days being forecasted, the nurse manager must estimate the acuity level of the patients to more accurately determine the level, competency, number, and mix of nursing personnel needed to care for those patients.

The definition of an FTE is a personnel standard that allows for measuring and planning the staffing budgets. An FTE is equal to 1 person working 8 hours a day, 5 days a week, 50 weeks a year (2080 hours). It can be expressed in decimals as 1.0 (full-time) or .5 (half-time). An FTE does not necessarily mean one person; it can be two, three, or four workers providing enough hours to represent one person working a full-time shift. Figure 7-4 provides an example of a personnel budget form.

CLASSIFICATION OF COSTS

Costs incurred in the delivery of a service or the making of a product are called total costs and may be either direct or indirect; variable or fixed. A solid understanding of the types of costs and how they relate to your unit will allow you to make more appropriate decisions on how to cut costs, determine break-even points, and measure the effectiveness of any action.

A cost center is any department or unit of the organization that has been designated as an area that accumulates operating costs. A nursing unit may have more than one cost center. More effective management can be accomplished by segregating costs and analyzing the benefits against the expenses.

Fixed Costs

A fixed cost is a cost that does not change with the level of volume (i.e., the number of patients). Mortgage, loan, and bond payments are examples of fixed costs. Certain departments are considered fixed cost, or overhead, departments, such as medical records, admitting, the business office, and administration.

Variable Costs

A variable cost is a cost that is associated only with a specific activity (i.e., supply costs). Dressing supplies are the only cost if a patient is being treated for a wound. Variable costs may go either up or down with census shifts and are the first to be analyzed when operations are being reviewed.

Direct Costs

Direct costs can be allocated directly to the making or delivery of an item or service (e.g., nursing care hours in an intensive care unit or supply costs).

Staff	(Productive and Nonproductive, exclude relief) POSITION SHIFTS								
Position Description	Position Class	AM	PM	NIGHT	1992 Total FTE	Annual holiday days accrual	Holiday percent replace	Average sick day usage	Sick percent replace
Position Description	Position Class	Vacation FTE	Holiday FTE	Sick FTE		Non-productive FTE			

FIG. 7-4   A personnel budget form.

Indirect Costs

Those costs associated with the provision of services, but which cannot be directly linked to one specific area or service, are indirect costs. Generally, these costs are spread over the entire organization or areas of the organization based on some approved allocation method. Some examples of these costs would be security costs, housekeeping, and utilities.

Budgets can be defined as both planning documents and control documents—two methods of ensuring financial viability in this dynamic marketplace. The margin for error is decreasing because reimbursement tightens while the cost of providing services increases

Educ/ orientaion days usage	Educ/ orientaion percent replace	Non- productive total days					Holiday over- time hours	Annual stand- by hours	Annual call- back hours
Relief FTE	Educ/ orientation FTE	Stand- by FTE	C/B FTE				Productive FTE	Total FTE	FTE Vari Productive STD

FIG. 7-4, cont'd   For legend see opposite page.

daily because of new technologies and equipment, as well as higher salary demands by all health care personnel.

THE ROLE OF THE NURSE MANAGER IN THE BUDGET PROCESS

Historically, nurse managers have not been perceived as astute financial managers. Their expertise was in the clinical area, and the expectation was that the finance department would worry about reimbursing the cost of providing nursing service. But for nurse managers to successfully participate in negotiations between all hospital departments vying for decreasing budget monies, they must speak the same language and understand fiscal processes. Nurse managers must also be able to enter into the budget process without personalizing any budgetary actions. Staff cutbacks are sometimes inevitable solutions to the daily decreases in reimbursement for care. Special programs or increases of staff members must sometimes wait until the financial outlook improves or revenues are generated to pay for those services.

To plan more realistically and effectively, a nurse manager must be organized and consistent during the budget planning process, anticipating all changes that may occur within the budgeted time frame.

Budget Assumptions: Getting Ready to Start

Initially, all departmental objectives and goals must be analyzed to give the nurse manager direction in allocating given resources.

New projects and added or deleted services must be taken into account, along with the ongoing service of the unit. Historical data about estimated patient days, levels of acuity, or types of patients are also needed to make a more educated budget estimate. Knowledge of equipment needs, physician requests, and regulatory requirements are also essential for proper budgeting.

It is important to note that *budgets as planning and controlling documents are only as reliable as the data that were used in the development of the plan.* Changing requirements, service levels, and/or charge structures may be revised, and the budget document may not be as relevant as it was when prepared. The nurse manager must be able to discern those changes which occur between development and implementation of the unit budget and reflect those changes properly once the budget period begins.

Recessionary cutbacks in tax revenues have forced certain state and local governments to reduce health care allocations immediately and across the board to all providers in their jurisdictions (e.g., California MediCal cuts and then their inability to pass a budget, thus resulting in the issuing of "warrants," or IOUs, for payment to health providers). Those health care entities with a large percentage of state Medicaid patients risk serious, if not fatal, financial duress if banking institutions refuse to accept the warrants as funds. Plans of action must be in place to meet such demands, including the issuance of loans or the reduction of services to stay financially viable.

The budget approval process is a dynamic function. Completed documents are submitted to higher management to be compiled and included in a larger document. For that reason, all department or service budgets are reviewed in relation to the prioritized needs of the organization.

BUDGET DECISIONS THAT MUST BE ADDRESSED

✔ Do the benefits justify the costs?

✔ Is the budget consistent with the hospital's strategic goals and objectives?

✔ Is the budget reasonable and realistic?

✔ Will the organization be able to support the budget?

Based on the organization's needs and financial abilities, a nurse manager may not receive all that has been requested during the budget process and thus must cut some costs from the budget. But the manager must be able to understand and distinguish the unit's core service and needs to more efficiently make the required cuts. Again, it is important that the new nurse manager not personalize any budget cuts because such behavior is counterproductive to successful management. Discussions should be ongoing between the unit managers and their senior management staff during the budget process to address the possibility of such problems.

BUDGETARY INDICATORS

Once settled in your new position as nurse manager with a basic understanding of the fiscal process, set up a financial report filing system that allows you the ability to monitor your unit's activities.

Following is a list of financial reports that are used in various organizations:

Unit Reports

Payroll report	Employee earnings and hours worked by pay period
Productivity report	Usually a percentage of total or productive hours worked for a given number of units of service (i.e., patient days as compared to budget)
Budget variance report	A listing of general ledger accounts, with monthly actual costs-to-budget amounts and cumulative year-to-date (CYTD) actual costs-to-budget amounts. Any deviance, whether positive or negative, is called a variance
Supply variance report	A listing by department of all supply costs and associated variances as compared with the budget amounts

All reports should be filed separately in chronologic order, with the most recent on top. If your institution produces computerized ledger reports, there are expandable notebooks used to store these documents. These should be stored by fiscal year or fiscal period for easy retrieval and review.

Variances

Review all reports to ensure they are complete and correct; report discrepancies immediately to your supervisor or finance office (per hospital policy). Variances should be analyzed quickly and discussed with your supervisor. Abnormal or negative trends are insidious in nature, and you must closely oversee this aspect of your operations to analyze such happenings and develop plans of action to correct identified negative trends.

Variances are the differences between the budgeted amounts and the actual amounts. Usually a negative ($-$) variance means a positive bottom line. In monitoring variances during periods of higher-than-budgeted volumes (i.e., numbers of patients), the manager must be aware of the forces of flexible versus fixed budgeting techniques. Variances may look askew, but when adjusted for volume, appear right on target.

For an example of a productivity report showing a personnel usage variance, see Figure 7-5. Different job classifications, as well as their corresponding productivity standards, are noted in the first two columns. The actual versus budgeted units of service for that pay period are noted in the third through the sixth columns. A negative number in the variance column notes less-than-anticipated units of service. The productive and nonproductive FTE blocks show the actual versus the budgeted amounts of personnel. However, these are fixed-budget figures and do not reflect the FTEs used as compared with the actual units of service.

In the total FTE block is a flexible budget figure. That figure determines the number of FTEs available based on the actual units of service. In other words, if your unit had budgeted 4 FTEs for 16 hours of service and only 12 hours of service were given, only 12 hours should have been used. If, in the above scenario, you had used only 3 FTEs, the productivity rating would have been 100%. If you used the full 4 FTEs (as your budget states), your productivity would be only 75%.

The two blocks in Figure 7-5 for productive and total hours per unit of service actually address the productivity standard used for your department. In the case of the ICU, the productive standard for ICU days would be 16.109 hours per day; the total standard would be 17.688 hours per day.

The salary variance of $3,115 denotes a loss of $3,115 during that pay period resulting from overstaffing the ICU by approximately 13% to 15%. The $3,115 is an average amount of dollars for personnel costs across the board in the hospital. It is used as a guide to denote in dollar amounts the loss the hospital incurs from staffing overages. The positive amounts, such as are noted in the laboratory and pulmonary function columns, show the amount of monies saved by increasing or decreasing staff.

Monitoring figures pay period by pay period allows the manager to review operations and identify negative trends. However, because of dramatic census shifts, labor contracts, and holiday and sick coverage, the manager must also look at the productivity rating over a longer period—either month to month or on a quarterly basis.

ASK QUESTIONS

Once you organize all the reports you have received to monitor the operations of your unit, set up a meeting with your fiscal repre-

Seaside Hospital
Productivity Report PPE: 6/20/92

Unit of Service					Productive FTE				Nonproductive FTE			Total FTEs	
Dept	Desc	Act	Bud	Var	Var%	Act	Bud	Var	Staff Var	Act	Bud	Var	Act	Fixed Budget
ICU	ICU DAYS	54	63	(9)	-15%	11.3	12.8	1.4	11%	2.4	1.3	-1.2	13.7	14.0
M/S	M/S DAYS	267	282	(15)	-5%	25.7	28.0	2.2	8%	3.9	3.1	-0.8	29.6	31.1
E.R.	ER VISITS	807	716	91	13%	14.0	13.3	-0.6	-5%	2.4	1.1	-1.3	16.4	14.4
O.R.	OR MINS	13,310	11,363	1,947	17%	14.7	11.6	-3.1	-26%	2.5	1.4	-1.1	17.2	13.0
NSG ADM	ADJ PD	813	895	(81)	-9%	6.7	5.5	-1.2	-22%	0.4	0.9	0.5	7.1	6.4
Home Health	H.H. VISITS	444	577	(133)	-23%	14.2	15.7	1.6	10%	0.7	2.0	1.3	14.8	17.7
Lab	TESTS	8119	7898	221	3%	13.7	13.2	-0.5	-4%	1.6	1.9	0.3	15.3	15.0
Pulm Func.	CAP UNITS	9,023	9,750	(727)	-7%	1.0	1.4	0.4	29%	0.1	0.1	0.0	1.1	1.5
Medical Records	ADJUSTED PT DAYS	813	895	(81)	-9%	7.1	6.1	-0.9	-15%	0.4	0.8	0.4	7.5	6.9

FIG. 7-5   A productivity report.

sentative. Ask questions and clarify statements or accounts at that time. Be clear as to the purpose of each report and what the data can tell you about the operations of your unit.

PRODUCTIVITY MEASUREMENT

Once approval has been given to the unit budget, the nurse manager must be able to abide by the financial constraints of that budget while still providing quality patient care services.

Total FTEs		Productive Hours/Unit of Service				Total Hours/Unit of Service					
Flex Budget	Flex Var	Act	Bud	Var	Var%	Act	Bud	Var	Var %	Salary Var	Pro%
11.9	−1.8	16.755	16.109	−0.646	−4%	20.310	17.688	−2.622	−15%	($3115)	87%
29.5	−0.2	7.707	7.939	.0232	3%	8.877	8.831	−0.046	−1%	($221)	99%
16.3	−0.1	1.387	1.490	0.104	7%	1.621	1.613	−0.008	−1%	($116)	99%
15.3	−1.9	0.088	0.082	−0.006	−8%	0.103	0.092	−0.012	−13%	($4357)	89%
5.8	−1.3	0.661	0.493	−0.168	−34%	0.696	0.572	−0.124	−22%	($2527)	82%
13.6	−1.2	2.551	2.179	−0.372	−17%	2.675	2.454	−0.220	−9%	($1663)	92%
15.4	0.1	0.135	0.133	−0.002	−1%	0.151	0.152	0.001	1%	$199	101%
1.4	0.31	0.009	0.012	0.003	27%	0.010	0.013	0.003	23%	$445	130%
6.3	−1.2	0.695	0.549	−0.146	−27%	0.734	0.618	−0.116	−19%	($1323)	84%

FIG. 7-5, cont'd　　For legend see opposite page.

Before development of the cost-containment and tight-reimbursement health care arena that has dominated the industry during the past decade, cost-based reimbursement did not stress the need to be productive and use scarce resources in an efficient manner.

Productivity has been measured in many industries, and standards have been developed that enable a manager to quantify the effectiveness of any staff. For a long time, the production of only goods, not services, was felt to warrant productivity measurement. The introduction of time-and-motion engineers into patient care units was not accepted well by staff members. The staff felt that nursing care could not be measured and that any constraint would be detrimental to the quality of the service delivered.

But economic survival forced productivity standards into the forefront of operational management techniques in health care settings. All activities of patient care were thoroughly examined and dissected to determine the amount or consumption of labor hours needed to provide that service. The average of all those hours were compiled to develop a patient care standard.

FINANCIAL STANDARDS

There are many types of standards: national, industrial, local, and institutional. A standard is developed for use in a manager's facility, and the forecasting, budgeting, and actual review of operations must be consistent with the productivity standard that was designed to monitor the work of that individual department.

If a manager wants to develop a departmental standard, the following criteria need to be examined and then calculated into an amount of time per patient care service. First, a standard of quality must be agreed on for a given service, and then the average amount of time necessary to complete that service would constitute the production standard. Various methods can be used to gain that information: (1) an actual time-and-motion study, (2) an average formulated over a given period for the same types of services, (3) historical data, or (4) an educated guess if there are no data available.

BREAK-EVEN ANALYSIS

In learning how to be efficient in the management of your unit, the ability to determine a break-even analysis is important. Generally, all services or products offered by a business should be able to show a profit or should at least break even on costs.

However, breaking even is not possible in some situations in hospitals, and the decision must be made whether to keep such services and balance their costs with other services. Such a costly service would be a trauma center or emergency service. Because of the specialized and expensive staff and equipment required to maintain the legal status of a trauma center on a 24-hour, 7-days-per-week basis, most facilities do not break even on this service. Most of the patients do not have sufficient insurance to cover all expenses, if they have insurance at all. However, it is a needed and vital service to the community.

Calculating Break-Even Points

The point at which the revenues equal the expenses is called the break-even point. A quick method to determine the break-even point is by dividing the fixed cost of a service by the contribution margin per unit of service (see the definition below of contribution margin). Break-even analysis is very important in a hospital because hospitals generally have very high fixed costs.

Budgetary Example in a Home Health Agency

For example, in a home health agency, the following information is given:

Monthly fixed costs:	$10,000
Revenue per visit:	$100
Direct cost per visit:	$50
Contribution margin per visit	$50

$$\text{Contribution margin} = \text{Revenue per visit} - \text{Direct cost per visit}$$

The break-even point (or the point at which the next unit of service's contribution margin is considered profit) would be:

$$\$10,000 \div \$50 = 200 \text{ visits}$$

Contribution Margin

The contribution margin is the amount of revenue left after the direct costs of providing the service are subtracted.

For example, the direct salary cost of a home health visit is $45 per visit, and the supply cost is $5, while the charge to the patient or payer is $100 per visit;

$$\text{Direct cost: } \$45 + \$5 = \$50$$

The contribution margin would be the difference between the revenue and the direct cost, or:

$$\$100 - \$50 = \$50$$

The contribution margin ($50) is then applied to the indirect, overhead, and/or administrative costs of doing business.

PRODUCTIVITY RATINGS

Productivity rating is measured as a percentage:

$$\text{Standard} \div \text{actual} = \underline{\quad} \%$$

For example, if the standard for a home care nurse is 2 hours per visit, and the payroll records reflect that the average hours per visit over a given time frame was 2.5 hours, the rating would be 80%. The usual variance is ±5%.

If the standard was 2 hours per visit and the nurse averaged 1.5 hours per visit, the rating would be 133%. That is a positive variance and reflects an overall savings to the home health agency.

FUTURE TRENDS

As the health care industry continues its reforms and integrates TQM and fiscal responsibility into its case management structure, patient outcomes should improve and become more predictable.

Large employers such as companies in the automobile industry, point out that they pay $300 to $500 of the revenue generated per new car for health care benefits for their employees. Just as consumers demand quality products off the automobile assembly line, health care consumers are demanding a standardized set of services that offer comparable outcomes.

This is a new concept to health providers—the argument has always been that health care is not quantifiable, as is the manufacturing sector of the economy. However, studies are showing that a wide divergence in standard practices for the same set of diagnoses or symptoms exists all across the country.

Large Business Groups on Health (LBGH, a lobbying group for business entities) is collecting and disseminating data on local hospitals and physician providers to the community denoting positive and adverse trends of service. LBGH is demanding that health care providers take a proactive stance for cost-effective, quality health care.

Once standards are clearly defined and routinely monitored, incentive systems can be put into place to reward those employees who use the best quality indicators, TQM, and patient satisfaction to turn their health care facility into a well-managed and effective organization.

Profit-sharing is a novel trend for health care, and it has been successfully integrated into a for-profit facility on the East Coast. It has inspired the staff to work more productively and to produce a better end result—a satisfied patient and physician.

SUMMARY

Health care finance is a complex and demanding field, and nurse managers are an essential link in maintaining cost-effective, quality-oriented care. By understanding the role of cost accounting in the planning, delivery, and evaluation of care, the nurse manager can provide the best advocacy for patient care services in health care .

Financial managers are usually trained in the accounting or finance fields and usually do not have the education or expertise to make patient care decisions that involve cutbacks or reductions in services. Their focus is on improving the hospital's bottom line and providing sound financial decisions.

Nurses with business acumen and finance knowledge blend the best of both worlds and provide the most equitable perception of the budgeting process. Always be aware of the forces that are affecting the delivery of your patient care and be able to adapt to new and challenging situations.

REFERENCES

1. Scholtes, PR et al: *The team handbook,* Madison, WI, 1989, Jointer Associates.
2. Shillinglaw, G, Meyer E: *Accounting: a management approach,* ed 7, Homewood, Ill, 1983, Richard D Irwin.
3. Anthony N, Reece J: *Accounting texts and cases,* ed 7, Homewood, Ill, 1983, Richard D Irwin.

Glossary of Financial Terminology

The following is a list of key financial terms that can be very helpful to you while learning your way as a new nurse manager.

Accounting   The process of identifying and measuring an economic variable. Managerial accounting refers to the information that is prepared to assist managers in making decisions on how to use limited resources effectively and efficiently.

Acuity level   A measured level that describes the severity of illness in patients by a weighted statistical method. Usually most acuity systems have four classifications of patients that describe the amount of time a nurse spends daily with each type of patient (i.e., ICU patients may have an acuity level of 4, denoting a 1:1 RN:patient ratio). It was calculated using formulas that measured nursing functions in terms of actual time.

Gross revenue/income   The total amount charged for a service.

Hours per patient day (HPPD)   The number of nursing care hours provided per patient per 24-hour day.

Liabilities   The financial obligations of the hospital or other health care organization (i.e., accounts payable or loan amounts).

Medicaid program   A state health insurance program for those individuals meeting certain financial guidelines which is supported by the federal government in association with funds from a given state. Not all states have Medicaid programs, and the programs and their coverage vary from state to state.

Medicare program   The federally funded health insurance program for those individuals over the age of 65 and/or disabled. It was started in 1965 and totally revolutionized the delivery of health care in the United States. It reimbursed hospitals and other health care providers on a cost-based system. The health care system then experienced rapid growth because there were no incentives built into the program to conserve and/or properly use resources.

Currently, the Medicare program is undergoing extensive scrutiny and revision to meet the growing needs of the burgeoning older population. Hospitals have been taken out of the cost-based system, and the prospective pay, or DRG, system has taken its place.

Medicare-certified home health agencies are still currently cost-based. Studies are being conducted to determine the best method to establish a prospective payment system for the rapidly growing home care industry in the near future.

Net income   The difference between the gross revenue and what remains after all expenses have been deducted.

Nonproductive hours   Paid hours that are not associated with the provision of care or service (i.e., vacation, sick, and education leave).

Patient classification system   A system to classify patients using different criteria sets. The goal of the patient classification system is to allocate nursing personnel to specific units (i.e., staffing matrix).

Productive hours   Paid hours that are associated with provision of care or service, including regular time, overtime, and holiday time.

Relative value units   A numerical value that has been coded to reflect the relative complexity of a given service, such as time, skill, and overhead costs for a certain procedure. Many third-party payers attach a dollar value to these units in calculating reimbursement rates. An example of a service measured in RVUs is rehabilitation services (physical therapy).

Staffing mix   The type and ratio of professional personnel (RNs) to other patient care personnel. This mix varies from hospital to hospital and is gaining in popularity as the need to decrease personnel costs becomes more evident.

Nurse extenders or licensed vocational/practical nurses in tandem with an RN are two examples of using a varied staffing mix. This is a move away from the all-RN staffs demanded by the nursing industry in the 1970s and 1980s.

CHAPTER 8

Legal Issues and Risk Management

Elizabeth Hogue

This chapter focuses the new nurse manager's attention on significant legal issues. Discussion of legal issues in nursing management could fill *several* books, and it is often difficult for the new nurse manager to know where to focus her attention in terms of legal issues. In addition, the new manager's difficulty in discerning significant legal issues may be further complicated by the staff's initial tendency to raise numerous questions or concerns about legal issues. In the absence of effective management, staff members may seek structure and stability in their work environment through the law. Once effective nursing leadership is in place, the tendency to see everything as a legal issue will disappear.

However, significant legal issues exist that always merit the attention of competent nurse managers. New managers should immediately focus their attention on these issues and continuously monitor developments in the following areas:

- Negligence
- Consent to treatment, including the patient's right to refuse treatment
- Employment issues

NEGLIGENCE

Health care providers often equate negligence with something going wrong. In fact, there are risks associated with treatment. Just because something goes wrong does not mean that any legal liability exists. Rather, there are four components that every patient must be able to prove were involved to show that nurses were negligent:

1. Duty
2. Breach
3. Causation
4. Injury

All four of these components must be involved to prove negligence. If patients fail to prove even one of these elements, they lose their cases. Thus these elements can serve as a checklist for the new nurse manager to use to manage risks and evaluate the likelihood of legal liability. If she can defeat even one of the components, no legal liability exists.

But a determination that there is no legal liability is certainly not all that should concern the nurse manager. Managers may have significant ethical, quality assurance, employment, and licensure concerns that should be pursued even when no legal liability exists. However, it is helpful to eliminate concerns about legal liability even when other serious considerations require resolution.

It is also important to remember that involvement of these elements constitutes the definition of negligence that is actually used by the courts. That is, when courts attempt to determine whether providers are negligent, they consider these elements in relation to each case to determine liability. This is true regardless of the state in which nurses provide care. The definition of negligence in New York is the same as in California. The legal definitions of duty, breach, causation, and injury are discussed below.

Duty

Duty is the obligation owed by providers to their patients. Thus the existence of a provider-patient relationship is a prerequisite to liability.

The duty owed by nurses to their patients is a duty of reasonable care. Of course, the key question then becomes: What is reasonable? The law says that what is reasonable is what other reasonably prudent nurses do under the same or similar circumstances. Nurses know what other nurses do by examining standards of care. Standards of care define nurses' duties to their patients. Sources of such standards of care are listed in the box on the next page.

SOURCES OF STANDARDS OF CARE

- The employer's internal policies and procedures
- Court decisions
- Standards of professional nursing organizations such as the American Nurses Association (ANA) and the National League for Nursing (NLN)
- State licensure statutes
- Requirements of third-party payors
- Standards of accreditation organizations such as the Joint Commission for the Accreditation of Healthcare Organizations (JCAHO)

The Importance of Policies and Procedures

Policies and procedures constitute perhaps the most important source for standards of care. Developing appropriate standards of care through policies and procedures is certainly a double-edged sword for nurse managers. Although it provides an opportunity to establish standards that are appropriate for institutions and staff members, the law requires strict adherence to these standards once they have been developed.

In addition, developing policies and procedures is an exceptionally tedious task for several reasons. First, some nurses believe that policies and procedures should cover every possible contingency associated with the policy subject. Nurses who share this belief want such policies so that they feel they have clear guidance. Other nurses, however, believe that policies and procedures should provide only broad guidance, within which nurses should exercise appropriate professional judgment. Obviously, finding a balance between these two competing goals is necessary. Policies that are too detailed often prove useless because staff members do not have the time or inclination to read through volumes to understand procedure. Conversely, promoting clarity of expectations of staff members is one of the basic tenets of effective nursing management.

Developing standards of care through policies and procedures is further complicated by the sheer number of individuals and committees that typically review a new or revised policy or procedure. Often, what goes into the process bears little resemblance to the final result.

Despite these obstacles, nurse managers must persist in developing and maintaining appropriate policies and procedures. A key to success is to avoid thinking that this process is ever complete. Nursing policies and procedures should be under almost constant review and scrutiny; they are not static. Rather, they change often because of experience, judgment, and new clinical developments.

KEY STEPS TO MANAGING RISK THROUGH POLICIES AND PROCEDURES

Specifically, nurse managers should follow the five key steps below.

✔ Review policies and procedures once every 3 months.

✔ Involve different staff members in reviewing policies and procedures so that various points of view are obtained and the staff has an opportunity to review standards of care.

✔ Make needed changes promptly.

✔ Ensure that all staff members are informed of changes in policies and procedures.

✔ Ensure that all new staff members read and understand the policies and procedures.

If nurse managers follow these steps, they will have greater assurance that they appropriately manage risk by careful definition of duty in terms of policies and procedures.

Breach

Nurses may breach their duty to patients by doing something they should not do, which is commonly referred to as an *act*. They may also fail to do something that they should do, which is often referred to as an *omission*. In many malpractice cases, patients are able to prove that providers committed more than one act or omission. Yet, they *need* prove only *one* act or omission to prove a breach.

For example, in one recent court case, a man was brought to the emergency room with a chest wound. He was evaluated to see if he needed a thoracic surgeon. It was determined that he did not have such a need. He was reevaluated an hour later, and it was determined that he, indeed, needed a thoracic surgeon. The surgeon was called but did not arrive for over an hour. On the surgeon's arrival, the patient was rushed into the operating room, where he died. The family sued, claiming that if the surgeon had arrived earlier, the patient would not have died. During the course of discovery, the attorney for the patient's family found an emergency room policy that stated that if the thoracic surgeon was called and did not arrive within 30 minutes, the patient must be transferred to another hospital. The family won this case because the nursing staff breached its duty as established in emergency room policies and procedures.

Causation

A patient must show that the act or omission of the nurse caused injury or damage. The best way to define causation is in terms of "but for." That is, but for the action or inaction of the provider, the patient would not have been injured. Another way to consider causation is in terms of what courts call "foreseeability." That is, if providers should have foreseen that their act(s) and/or omission(s) would cause injury or damage to a patient, the injury was foreseeable and therefore caused by providers. Conversely, if providers could not have foreseen that their act(s) and/or omission(s) would cause injury or damage to a patient, the injury was not foreseeable and therefore was not caused by providers.

Time is certainly a consideration with this requirement. For example, when a patient who is released from a mental health institution causes injury or damage to an individual after release, it is tempting to find a causal connection between the patient's release and the injuries sustained. Nurses recognize, however, that an individual's mental status may change very rapidly. Therefore no causal connection may exist whatsoever between release and the injuries.

Nurses sometimes ask how long of a period must elapse before causation is no longer a concern. This period varies depending on the circumstances of individual cases. Providing specific rules is thus impossible. A good general rule is that the longer the period between the providers' action or inaction and the occurrence of the injury, the less likely that providers will be held liable.

Injury

To be held liable, nurses must injure or damage their patients. Most of the time the courts insist on a physical injury to establish liability. Courts require proof of physical injury for several reasons. First, if the alleged injury is not physical, patients may be faking their injuries. Courts have evidentiary requirements that must be met to prove injury. If the claimed injury is mental or emotional in nature, it is almost impossible to prove. Second, the courts recognize that a certain amount of irritation and inconvenience simply accompany being alive. It is not the job of the courts to address all of these inconsequential irritations and inconveniences. Rather, individuals are generally required to accept life's daily aggravations that are relatively insignificant. Unless patients can show a physical injury, their complaints may fall into the category of mere irritation and inconveniences, not legal liability. Finally, judges are increasingly distressed about their overcrowded dockets. In many jurisdictions there are so many cases pending that it takes several years for a civil, noncriminal case to come to trial. Courts recognize that caseloads will increase many times over if they start considering cases involving claims for emotional injuries only. They therefore normally insist the claimant have a physical injury before they will find providers liable.

Extreme and Outrageous Behavior

The one exception to this general rule occurs when the behavior of providers is what the courts call "extreme and outrageous." Extreme and outrageous behavior is outside of the acceptable bounds of civilized behavior. Extreme and outrageous conduct is illustrated by the case in which a woman was in the delivery room about to deliver a baby. Her husband was with her at her head. She died precipitously. The father rushed around to his deceased wife's side and put his hand on her abdomen. He could feel the infant still moving. He turned to the delivery room staff and asked them to perform an emergency caesarean section to save the life of the infant. The staff refused. He stood in the delivery room, begging and pleading with the staff, until the infant died.

In this case, there may have been liability for the death of the mother. Certainly there was liability for the death of the infant. But the court also acknowledged liability directly related to the father, even though his injuries were emotional only. The court did not require a physical injury because it was clear that the father was not faking emotional injury in view of the circumstances. The court was also certain that the father's injuries amounted to more than mere irritation and inconvenience. Finally, even though court dockets are crowded, the courts are extremely interested in hearing this type of case because of the egregious conduct of the providers.

Thus, unless physical injury exists or extreme and outrageous conduct on the part of providers occurs, there is no legal liability. The focus of appropriate risk management is therefore on avoiding injuring patients. Good risk management truly amounts to damage control.

Nurse managers continually struggle to avoid certain common types of liability for negligence. They must work hard to control risk related to the following.

FIVE COMMON TYPES OF NEGLIGENCE

✔ Failure to properly monitor and observe patients.

✔ Improper diagnosis, particularly meningitis in pediatric patients, and myocardial infarctions.

✔ Falls.

✔ Foreign objects left in patients during surgery.

✔ Negligent premature discharge.

Negligent Premature Discharge

Negligent premature discharge, a relatively new area of potential liability for negligence, merits special attention. Concerns about negligent premature discharge are directly related to changes in the activities of third-party payors. Third-party payors now command the authority of providers with their assumed decision-making authority regarding patient care. Whereas providers previously made decisions regarding patient care, payors are now the gatekeepers to the health care delivery system. In view of this change, providers have begun to question why they may be held liable for the results of payment decisions of payors.

In response, payors argue that they do not write orders, including discharge orders. Providers are free to render as much care as they determine patients need. Payors are saying only that they will not pay for such care. Further, payors argue that, in many instances, they are simply enforcing a contract of insurance. Once benefits required by the contract have been provided, they are under no obligation to pay for additional care, regardless of the clinical condition of patients.

Providers, however, recognize the reality of the health care delivery system today, which is that payment decisions are, in essence, treatment decisions. Courts are considering the question raised by this reality to determine if payors should be held responsible for the injuries or damages that result from payors' adverse payment decisions. To date, three court decisions have addressed this issue.

Wickline versus The State of California

In the 1987 case of *Wickline versus The State of California*,[1] Mrs. Wickline had vascular disease. She had surgery, followed by a complicated recovery. Her physician wanted to keep her in the hospital to observe her for further complications. The Medicaid program, however, determined that no further payments would be made for acute care.

Mrs. Wickline's physician asked the Medicaid program for an additional extension of payment for acute care. Specifically, he asked the Medicaid program to pay for 8 additional days of care. Medicaid agreed to pay for 4 additional days.

At the end of the 4 days, the physician took no further action, and Mrs. Wickline went home. She developed further complications that ultimately resulted in the amputation of one of her legs. She then sued the Medicaid program. She claimed that the program had a duty to her to make payment for needed care that was breached when payment was refused for additional acute care. Medicaid's adverse payment decision, claimed Mrs. Wickline, caused injury to her in the form of the amputation of her leg.

It is important to note that there were alternatives that could have been used to limit risk in this case. For example, home care might have been an appropriate way to continue to monitor Mrs. Wickline for additional complications outside of the acute care setting. Even if nurse managers cannot ensure payment for the type or length of care that they regard as most desirable, it is important to arrange for other available care that may help to limit risk.

The court considered Mrs. Wickline's claim against the Medicaid program. It first recognized a so-called "changed reality" in the health care delivery system. That is, the court acknowledged that payors now make treatment decisions. Therefore, said the court, payors should be liable for adverse payment decisions that harm patients. The one condition placed on this shift of liability from providers to payors was that providers must satisfy what the court called "duty to protest." In other words, the Court said that providers would not be liable for results of adverse payment decisions so long as they protest payment decisions that they think will injure patients.

Because the physician in Mrs. Wickline's case did not protest the decision to terminate payment after the additional 4 days, the court did not find the Medicaid program liable in this case. The physician was not liable either because he was not a defendant in the case. The court made it clear, however, that from then on it would hold payors liable if they persisted in adverse payment decisions in view of protests by providers.

Valro versus Blue Cross and Blue Shield of Michigan

In the case of *Valro versus Blue Cross and Blue Shield of Michigan*,[2] workers at General Motors (GM) Company decided that they wanted more mental health and substance abuse benefits. GM agreed to provide the additional benefits but wanted to self-insure for them because these benefits can be expensive to offer.

GM went to Blue Cross and Blue Shield of Michigan and asked Blue Cross to run a pilot program to assist in developing these benefits. Blue Cross agreed. Both parties signed an agreement that, among other factors, made it clear that the pilot program would include a rigorous utilization review (UR). It would include preauthorization, precertification, concurrent review, and prospective and retrospective review.

Blue Cross then signed agreements with individual mental health providers to treat patients in the pilot program. All of the participants were satisfied until the UR program became so rigorous that it interfered with the providers' ability to deliver patient care or receive payments for providing care. They thought that the activities of Blue Cross amounted to the practice of medicine and sued them.

The court considered the providers' claims. In the court's view, the providers were simply attempting to ensure payment for fulfilling their ethical and legal duty to provide care to patients. The court came very close to calling them greedy wimps and termed the basis of the providers' law suit "strange stuff" on which to base a claim.

Thus the decision in the *Valro* case is inconsistent with that in the *Wickline* case. Specifically, *Wickline* says that providers are not required to treat patients if payment is denied, and, when patients are injured as a result, payors, not providers, are liable if payment is denied despite the providers' protests. *Valro*, however, says that providers have a legal and ethical obligation to provide care whether or not they receive payment.

Wilson versus Blue Cross and Blue Shield of Southern California et al

In the case of *Wilson versus Blue Cross and Blue Shield of Southern California, et al*,[3] decided in 1990, Mr. Wilson was hospitalized in Los Angeles for depression and anorexia. His physician, Dr. Taft, recommended in-patient care for 3 to 4 weeks. This recommendation was conveyed to Blue Cross.

Blue Cross contracted with a utilization review organization, Western Medical Review, to consider whether payment for claims such as Mr. Wilson's should be authorized. Dr. Wasserman at Western Medical Review considered Mr. Wilson's claim. He determined that he would authorize payment for the few days of inpatient care, which Mr. Wilson had already received but would not authorize payment for any additional inpatient care.

This decision was relayed to Dr. Taft and Mr. Wilson. Mr. Wilson had no other way to pay for his care and was discharged from the hospital.

Within the period during which Mr. Wilson probably would have been hospitalized, if his request for inpatient care had been authorized, he committed suicide. His parents then sued Blue Cross, Western Medical Review, and Dr. Wasserman, claiming that Mr. Wilson was negligently prematurely discharged as a result of the adverse payment decision.

The case was dismissed at the trial level based partly on Dr. Taft's failure to protest the adverse payment decision. On appeal, the court said that the previous ruling in the *Wickline* case was wrong. That is, payors are liable for the adverse payment decisions made that injure patients, whether or not providers protest these adverse payment decisions. This determination may serve as a useful precedent, permiting courts in other jurisdictions to reach a similar conclusion that payors are now liable for injuries that occur because of failure to pay for needed care.

In view of these court decisions, which are clearly inconsistent in some respects, nurse managers may well ask how to take appropriate action. The best advice at this time is to fulfill the duty to protest adverse payment decisions. This recommendation is based on the conclusion that such protests are good risk management. It is also based on the importance of the nurse's role as a patient advocate. If nurses do not speak for patients in the face of adverse payment decisions, it is unlikely that anyone will do so. Most patients do not understand the complex health care delivery system well enough to be their own advocates.

Nurse managers must be prepared to monitor developments in the area of liability for premature discharge. The last word has by no means been spoken on this important issue by courts and legislatures.

INFORMED CONSENT

Informed consent is not required for routine or emergency treatment. Routine care often includes physical examinations and drawing blood. Emergency treatment usually occurs when danger to life or permanent injury to patients' limbs is threatened.

Informed consent is required for treatment that is neither routine nor provided in response to an emergency. Generally, the need for valid informed consent increases in direct proportion to the risk of the treatment.

Prerequisites

The following two prerequisites must be met to obtain valid informed consent:

1. The patient must have the capacity to give consent in terms of chronologic age and the ability to understand information.
2. The patient's consent must be voluntary.

Generally, patients must be of legal age before they can consent to treatment. The age at which an individual is legally considered to be an adult varies from state to state but is usually at either age 18 or age 21. Exceptions to this requirement include:

- Minors who are emancipated because they are married, have borne a child, or are economically independent—the laws on this category vary from state to state.
- Minors who seek treatment for certain types of conditions such as sexually transmitted diseases, mental illness, or substance abuse—laws regarding these exceptions also vary from state to state.

Patients must also be able to understand information to give valid consent. Generally, this requirement means that they must be able to understand the consequences of their choices regarding treatment. Patients who have been found to be incompetent by the courts clearly lack capacity to understand information. Patients who have not been declared incompetent may, nonetheless, lack the necessary level of mental capacity. The best method for evaluating capacity is to use a mental status exam and to document the results in patients' records just before obtaining informed consent.

You should note that the law recognizes that capacity (the ability to understand information) may vary from moment to moment. Confused patients may suddenly seem much more lucid. It is appropriate to seek informed consent during such moments. Consent under such conditions is valid even after the patient becomes incapacitated once again.

A patient's consent must be voluntary (i.e., there can be no fraud or duress). Providers cannot tell patients that they are going to perform one treatment and actually perform an entirely different treatment. Providers walk a fine line between informing patients of the consequences of their refusal of treatment and threatening them.

INFORMATION NEEDED FOR INFORMED CONSENT

Patients who satisfy the prerequisites for informed consent must receive the following information:

✔ Description of the proposed treatment.

✔ Possible benefits of the proposed treatment.

✔ Significant risks associated with the treatment.

✔ Description of alternative treatments.

✔ A clear acknowledgement of their right to refuse treatment.

A description of the proposed treatment is essential because consent is valid only when a patient understands the treatment to be received. A patient cannot provide valid consent to a treatment that he or she does not understand.

Benefits of proposed treatment must never be described in absolute terms or as guarantees of results. If benefits are presented to patients as guarantees, a contract may be created that is breached by providers if they fail to deliver the promised result. Providers must speak of *possible* benefits from proposed treatment.

A provider is not required to share *all* risks with patients. Rather, a provider is required to share those risks which are either statistically significant or are especially important to patients in the provider's opinion. For example, if proposed surgery involves even a slight possibility of injury to a violinist's hands, this risk must be disclosed.

Alternative treatments must also be described. These may include medications, physical therapy, surgery, diet and exercise, or whatever could be of benefit to the patient.

Finally, the unqualified right of patients to refuse any treatment must be acknowledged as part of the process of obtaining informed consent. Providers should make a clear statement to this effect, which should be specifically acknowledged by patients.

Patients who consent to treatment after the prerequisites have been met and the above information has been given have given valid informed consent. Verbal consent is acceptable.

It is important, however, to document the patient's consent. Providers use several methods to accomplish this goal. The most popular vehicle is undoubtedly a consent form, which is useful only when it documents the specific information given to the patient. Other providers use progress notes summarizing the consent process. Audio and video recordings are also acceptable means of documenting informed consent.

Nurse managers should understand that it is the physician's job to obtain valid informed consent. Nurses may ask patients to sign forms documenting that they have given informed consent. Their signature on such forms as witnesses means that they saw the patient sign the form; their signature does not verify that patients received appropriate information. But nurse managers must also realize that the nursing staff has a vested interest in making sure informed consent is obtained because health care is almost always provided as a team. When one member of the team fails to perform or to adequately protect the team, the whole team is at risk, not just one member.

Suppose, however, that patients cannot meet the prerequisites of informed consent because they lack capacity either because of chronologic age or lack of ability to understand information. Who may give substitute consent on behalf of such patients?

THOSE WHO CAN GIVE SUBSTITUTE CONSENT ON BEHALF OF PATIENTS

✔ Parents on behalf of minors. In the case of separation or divorce, either the custodial or the noncustodial parent may consent unless he or she is prohibited from doing so in a separation agreement or a divorce decree. Nurse managers should educate staff to obtain copies of relevant documents and to place copies of these documents on patients' charts to certify that appropriate individuals gave consent on behalf of minors.

✔ Courts.

✔ Guardians of the person. Courts appoint two types of guardians or conservators: guardians of the property and guardians of the person. Only guardians of the person may consent to health care. Staff must obtain a copy of any decree of guardianship and place it on the patient's chart to document valid informed consent.

✔ Attorneys-in-fact. Attorneys-in-fact are appointed to act on behalf of patients in powers of attorney. Powers of attorney are very flexible instruments. Nurses must therefore obtain a copy of any power of attorney under which an individual claims authority to evaluate the scope of their powers. Powers of attorney may be executed only by patients who have mental capacity. When patients become permanently mentally incapacitated, it is too late to sign a power of attorney. Durable powers of attorney survive the incapacity of patients. The laws governing powers of attorney vary from state to state.

✔ State statutes. Some states have passed laws that permit individuals to make decisions regarding health care in the absence of a guardian or attorney-in-fact. There is significant variation among the state statutes.

WITHHOLDING AND WITHDRAWING TREATMENT
No Code Orders

"No Code" or "Do Not Resuscitate" orders are a form of withholding treatment. It is important for nurse managers to understand, however, that these orders permit providers to withhold *only* treatment related to resuscitation if patients need such measures. Such orders do not apply to withholding nourishment, hydration, or IV fluids.

No code orders may be entered by physicians at their discretion for terminally ill patients after consultation with competent patients or family members. Physicians are required to provide these orders.

No code orders may not be transferred between institutions. Patients who had no code orders in long-term care facilities must have a new order entered when admitted to a hospital.

Some institutions permit partial no code orders. Partial no code orders are undesirable from an administrative point of view. It is extremely difficult for staff members to remember what each patient's no code order permits.

Verbal No Code Orders

There is a clear difference of opinion regarding verbal no code orders. The best practice appears to permit them only under the following circumstances:

- They are given in the presence of two witnesses.
- They are valid for a very limited period before a written order is required, preferably 24 to 48 hours.

Withholding Other Forms of Treatment

Withholding or withdrawing other forms of treatment is always acceptable if the decision is made by competent adult patients. Difficulties arise, however, when family members or next of kin want to make decisions regarding withholding or withdrawing treatment. The question is: Under what circumstances may treatment be withheld from patients who lack capacity?

First, the providers must make a determination that the patient is either terminally ill or in a persistent vegetative state. This determination should be documented in the chart.

The question then becomes who can make decisions on behalf of the patient. The most important court decision that addressed this issue was *Cruzan versus Director, Missouri Department of Health,*[4] a 1990 decision of the U.S. Supreme Court. In this case a young woman, Nancy Cruzan, was in an automobile accident. When rescue personnel reached the scene, Ms. Cruzan had no pulse or respiration. These two essential functions were restored at the scene of the accident, and she was transported to a local hospital. The initial diagnosis was cerebral contusions compounded by significant lack of oxygen. Neurologists determined that Ms. Cruzan had probably been deprived of oxygen for approximately 12 to 14 minutes.

She remained in a coma for several weeks and then progressed to a semiconscious state. She was able to take some nourishment. To ensure proper nourishment and hydration, however, physicians asked her husband for permission to insert a gastrostomy tube. Her husband gave consent and the tube was implanted.

Despite valiant efforts, Ms. Cruzan remained in a vegetative state. That is, her body functioned almost entirely by its internal controls. It was able to maintain temperature, heartbeat, pulmonary ventilation, digestive activity, and reflex activity of muscles and nerves, which permits low-level conditioned responses. But she exhibited no behavioral evidence of self-awareness or awareness of her surroundings.

She remained in this state for several years. When it appeared unlikely that Ms. Cruzan would regain her mental capacity, her parents asked the hospital to remove the gastrostomy tube and to stop nourishment. Hospital personnel refused the request. Her parents filed suit and the case was eventually heard by the U.S. Supreme Court.

The Court said that each state has the right to safeguard the process for making decisions regarding withholding or withdrawing treatment. Each state is free to require whatever evidence it desires to accomplish this goal.

The Court recognized that family members do not always act in the best interest of patients. Therefore each state may decide to refuse to permit family members to make decisions on behalf of incompetent patients unless substantial proof shows that the decision made is one that the patient would also make. Substantial proof of patients' wishes may be expressed in durable powers of attorney or living wills.

Thus it is important for nurse managers to recognize that the requirements of the state in which they practice are paramount. At the extreme, states can refuse to permit withholding or withdrawing of treatment unless there is a clear statement from patients themselves about their wishes in the event of terminal illness or a persistent vegetative state.

To encourage clarity regarding patients' wishes, Congress passed the Patient Self-Determination Act, which became effective on December 1, 1991. This Act requires providers to obtain information from patients about their wishes regarding future health care. Such information is commonly called an *advance directive*. Specifically, providers must:

- Develop written policies and procedures to implement patients' rights to make decisions concerning future health care through the use of durable powers of attorney and/or living wills (advance directives) as permitted by state laws
- Provide all adult patients with written information about their rights under the laws of the state in which care is provided, including the right to consent to or refuse treatment, the right to sign advance directives, and a statement of the provider's policies governing implementation of patients' wishes
- Document in patients' files whether they have executed advance directives
- Provide education for all nursing staff members regarding advance directives

Compliance with this statute will undoubtedly assist nurse managers in clarifying issues of withholding and withdrawing treatment.

EMPLOYMENT

Regardless of practice setting, health care is a labor-intensive business. New nurse managers may feel lost in a maze of employment-related laws and court decisions, particularly those relating to discrimination and termination of the employment relationship. Two key questions are as follows:

1. How can the new nurse manager avoid discrimination against workers?
2. Under what circumstances may workers be terminated?

DISCRIMINATION

As most nurse managers already know, both federal and state laws prohibit discrimination on the basis of race, sex, handicapping condition, and religion. The following practical steps will help nurse managers ensure they do not violate these laws:

> ✔ Identify the essential job functions of all positions for which they are responsible. "Essential job functions" is a technical term. New nurse managers may need assistance from their HR departments to identify essential job functions and put them in writing in the form of job descriptions.
>
> ✔ Accept that reasonable accommodations are required so that individuals can perform essential job functions if the need for modifications is in any way related to a handicapping condition.
>
> ✔ Carefully follow the written essential job functions in carrying out all personnel activities, including hiring, evaluations, promotions, transfers, disciplinary actions, and terminations.
>
> ✔ Document all personnel actions in terms of the essential job functions.

New nurse managers who follow these guidelines will be successful at managing issues of employment discrimination.

Unlawful Termination

Similar steps may be taken to avoid liability for unlawful termination of workers who are not governed by a union contract. Generally, in the absence of any kind of contract, nurses can be hired and fired at will. Nurses are generally so-called "at-will" employees. Employees' attorneys have tested the absolute nature of this doctrine in recent years. Nurse managers may unwittingly fall into the trap of taking action that amounts to the creation of a contract without realizing that they have done so, thereby destroying their ability to terminate employees.

FIVE GUIDELINES TO HELP IN AVOIDING LIABILITY FOR UNLAWFUL TERMINATION OF EMPLOYEES

✔ Employee handbooks and policies and procedures must contain clear, unequivocal statements that they do not create a contract of employment.

✔ Managers must strictly adhere to their own policies and procedures, including definitions of circumstances that warrant immediate termination of employment.

✔ Except when immediate termination is warranted, managers must discipline workers progressively. They must first counsel workers, including development of specific corrective action before taking more serious action.

✔ Managers must thoroughly document all disciplinary action, especially counseling and corrective action.

✔ Consistency in following procedures and applying rules to all employees is essential.

Although it is often difficult to find the time and energy to follow these steps, they are vital to avoiding personnel problems.

SUMMARY

The information in this chapter is by no means exhaustive. There is much more for the new nurse manager to learn in the area of legal issues and readers are encouraged to seek further information when issues with legal implications arise. A glossary of legal terms is included in the appendix of this chapter for the reader's information.

But new managers who arrive at their offices on the first day in their new positions with no more than the information provided in this chapter are well on their way to success in managing the various risks associated with managing nursing personnel. This can be accomplished by remembering to:

1. Continuously monitor the quality of patient care to limit legal liability.

2. Assist patients in giving valid informed consent and making decisions regarding withholding and withdrawal of treatment.
3. Identify essential job functions and apply them in relation to all personnel functions, discipline employees progressively, and avoid creating contractual obligations unless you intend to do so.

REFERENCES

1. *Wickline v State of California,* 192 Cal App 3d 1630, 239 California Reporter 810, 1986.
2. *Valro v Blue Cross and Blue Shield,* 708 F Sup 826, ED Michigan, 1989.
3. *Wilson v Blue Cross of Southern California,* Cal App 2d, 271 California, Reporter 876, 1990.
4. *Cruzan v Harmon,* 760 S W 2d 408, Missouri 1988, en banc, *aff'd sub nom Cruzan v Director, Missouri Department of Health,* 110 S Ct 2841, 1990.

Glossary of Legal Terms

The author relied heavily on *Black's law dictionary*, ed 5, St. Paul, Minn, 1979, West Publishing, to prepare this glossary. Readers should make further use of this excellent resource when necessary.

Actual damages   Compensation for actual injuries or losses such as medical expenses or lost wages.

Affidavit   A written statement of facts given voluntarily under oath.

Allegation   The written statements by a party to a suit concerning what the party expects to prove.

Amended complaint   A corrected or revised version of the document filed in court by the plaintiff to being a suit.

Amicus curiae   Literally, "friend of the court." Person or oganizations with a strong interest in or views on a suit may ask the court in which the suit is filed for permission to file a brief to suggest a resolution of the case consistent with their views. *Amicus curiae* briefs are often filed in appeals of cases involving a broad public interest such as civil rights cases.

Appellant   The party who appeals the decision of one court to another court.

Appellate brief   Written arguments by attorneys required to be filed with an appellate court stating the reasons why the trial court acted correctly (appellee's brief) or incorrectly (appellant's brief). The contents and form of appellate briefs are often prescribed by the rules of various court systems. Appellate briefs usually contain a statement of issues presented for review by the appellate court, a statement of the case, argument, and a conclusion stating the precise action sought by the party submitting the brief.

Appellate review   Examination of a previous proceeding.

Appellee The party in a case against whom an appeal is brought. Sometimes also called the "respondent."

Assault Any conduct that creates a reasonable apprehension of being touched in an injurious manner. No actual touching is required to prove assault.

Assumption of the risk A defense to plaintiffs' claims based on the theory that plaintiffs may not recover for injuries to which they consent. To prove that the plaintiff assumed the risk, the defendant must show that: (1) the plaintiff had knowledge of a dangerous condition, (2) the plaintiff appreciated the nature or extent of the danger, and (3) the plaintiff voluntarily exposed himself or herself to the danger.

Attorney in fact Any person authorized by another to act in his or her place either for a particular purpose or for the transaction of business affairs in general. This authority is conferred by a document called a power of attorney.

Battery An unconsented, actual touching that causes injury.

Borrowed servant rule A theory of liability or negligence that is used to extend liability beyond the person who actually committed negligent acts to include those who had the right of control over the negligent actions.

Brief A written statement prepared by an attorney arguing a case in court. A brief contains a summary of the facts of the case, the pertinent laws, and an argument of how the law applies to the facts supporting an attorney's position.

Burden of proof The requirement of proving facts in dispute on an issue raised between the parties in a case.

Captain of the ship doctrine This doctrine imposes liability on surgeons in charge of operations for negligence of assistants during periods when those assistants are under the surgeons' control, even though the assistants are also employees of a hospital. This doctrine extends the borrowed servant rule to the operating rooms of hospitals.

Cause of action The fact or facts that give a person the right to begin a suit.

Common law As opposed to laws created by legislatures, the common law consists of legal principles based solely on usages and customs from time immemorial, particularly the ancient, unwritten laws of England.

Complaint   The first document filed in court by the plaintiff to begin a suit.

Conservator   Any individual appointed by a court to manage the affairs of an incompetent person.

Continuance   Adjournment or postponement of a session, hearing, trial, or other proceeding to a subsequent day or time.

Contributory negligence   A defense to a claim of negligence. Any act or omission on the part of the complaining party amounting to a breach of the duty the law imposes on everyone to protect themselves from injury that contributes to the injury complained of by the plaintiff.

Counterclaim   Claim presented by a defendant in opposition to the claim of the plaintiff. If the defendant establishes his claim, it will defeat or diminish the plaintiff's claim.

Cross-complaint   A defendant or cross-defendant (plaintiff) may file a cross-complaint based on (1) any claim against any of the parties who filed the complaint against him or her *or* (2) any claim against a person alleged to be liable whether or not the person is already a party to the suit. The claims in a cross-complaint must (1) arise out of the same transaction or occurrence as the original suit *and* (2) must make a claim or assert a right or interest in the property or the controversy that is the basis for the claim already made.

Cross-defendants   Plaintiffs who, subsequent to suing defendants, are then countersued by the defendants. Defendants in a suit brought by defendants.

Cross-examination   The questioning of a witness by an adverse party to test the truth of his or her testimony or to further develop it.

Declaratory judgment   Provided for in state and federal statutes. A person may seek a declaratory judgment from a court if there is an actual controversy among the parties, and the party asking for the declaratory judgment has some question or doubt about his or her legal rights. The judgment is binding on the parties both presently and in the future.

Defendant   The person defending or denying; the party against whom a civil lawsuit is brought or the accused in a criminal case.

Defense   A response to the claims of the other party stating the reasons why the claims should not be recognized.

Demurrer An argument in which the defendant admits the facts in the plaintiff's complaint, but claims that the facts are insufficient to require a response.

Deposition Advice by which one party asks oral questions of the other party or of a witness for the other party before the trial begins. The person who answers questions is called a deponent. The deposition is conducted under oath outside of the courtroom, usually in one of the lawyer's offices. A transcript, or word-for-word account, is made of the deposition.

Directed verdict When the party with the burden of proof fails to prove all necessary elements of the case, the trial judge may direct a verdict in favor of the other party because there can only be one result anyway.

Docket A list or calendar of cases to be tried during a particular period prepared by employees of the court for use by the court and attorneys.

Due process clause Two clauses in the United States Constitution, one in the Fifth Amendment applicable to the United States government, the other in the Fourteenth Amendment that protects persons from actions by the states. There are two aspects: (1) procedural, in which a person is guaranteed fair procedures, and (2) substantive, which protects a persons' property from unfair governmental interference. Similarly, clauses are in most state constitutions.

Due process of law An orderly proceeding in which a person receives notice of the proceeding and the subject matter of the proceeding and is given an opportunity to be heard and to enforce and protect his or her rights before a court or person(s) with power to hear and determine the case.

Equal protection clause A provision in the Fourteenth Amendment to the United States Constitution that requires every state to treat individuals in similar circumstances the same in terms of rights and redress of improper actions against them.

Ex parte On one side only; by or for one party; done for, on behalf of, or on the application of, one party only. A judicial proceeding, order, or injunction is *ex parte* when it is granted at the request of and for the benefit of one party only without notice to any person adversely interested.

False imprisonment A tort that consists of intentionally confining a person without his consent.

Felony   A crime of a more serious nature. Under federal law and many state statutes, a felony is any offense punishable by imprisonment for a term exceeding 1 year or by death.

Guardian   Any person responsible for managing the property of and protecting the rights of another person who, because of youth or lack of understanding, is incapable of managing his or her own affairs.

Guardian ad litem   A special guardian appointed by a court to prosecute or defend, on behalf of a minor or incompetent person, a suit to which the minor or incompetent person is a party.

Harmless error   Any trivial error or an error that is merely academic because it did not affect important rights of any party to a case and did not affect the final result of the case. Harmless error will not serve as a basis for changing a decision of the court.

Implied consent   Signs, actions or facts, or inaction or silence that indicate that consent is given.

In loco parentis   In the place of a parent; instead of a parent; charged with a parent's rights, duties, and responsibilities.

Infliction of emotional distress   Conduct going beyond that usually tolerated by society that is calculated to cause mental distress *and* that actually causes severe mental distress.

Informed consent   A person's agreement to allow something to happen that is based on a full disclosure of facts needed to make the decision intelligently.

Intent   Design, resolve, or determination that serves as the basis for a person's actions. Intent can rarely be proven directly but may be inferred from the circumstances.

Interrogatories   A tool to elicit information important to a case before trial. Interrogatories are written questions about the case submitted by one party to another party or witness. The answers to interrogatories are usually given under oath (i.e., the person answering the questions signs a sworn statement that the answers are true).

Judge a quo   Literally, "from which." A judge of a court from which a case was taken before a decision is made.

Judgment of nonsuit A decision by a court against plaintiffs when they are unable to prove their cases or refuse or neglect to proceed to trial. A court decision that leaves the issues undetermined.

Judgment notwithstanding the verdict (inov) A judgment entered by order to the court for a party, even though the jury decided in favor of the other party. A motion for directed verdict must usually be made before a judgment, notwithstanding the verdict.

Jurisdiction The right and power of a court to decide a particular case.

Jury instructions Statements made by the judge to the jury regarding the law applicable to the case the jury is considering that the jury is required to accept and apply. Attorneys for both sides usually furnish the judge with suggested instructions.

Justiciable controversy Courts will decide only justiciable controversies. That is, courts will decide only cases in which there is a real, substantial difference of opinion between the parties as opposed to a hypothetical difference or dispute or one that is academic or moot.

Leave to amend Permission or authorization given by a judge to any party to a suit to correct or reverse any document filed by the party with the court.

Locality rule To show negligence according to the locality rule, a plaintiff must prove that the defendant practitioner failed to render care considered reasonable in the same or in a similar geographical location.

Misdemeanor Criminal offenses less serious than a felony and usually punished by a fine or imprisonment in other than a penitentiary. Any criminal offense other than a felony.

Motion for new trial Request to a judge to set aside a decision already made in a case and to order a new trial on the basis that the first decision was improper or unfair.

Motion for summary judgment An application made to a court or judge to obtain a ruling or order that all or part of the other party's claim or defense should be eliminated from further consideration. This motion is made when a party believes there is no significant disagreement concerning important facts among the parties *and* the law supports the position of the party making the motion. A motion for summary judgment may be directed toward all or part of a claim or defense. It may be made on the basis of the pleadings or other portions of the record in the case, or it may be supported by affidavits and a variety of outside material.

Motion to dismiss An application made to a court or judge to order that the plaintiff's suit be eliminated from further consideration by the court or judge. This motion is usually made before a trial is held and may be based on a variety of reasons; for example, insufficiency of the plaintiff's claims or improper service of process of the plaintiff's suit on the defendant.

Motion to intervene/Plea in intervention A written request to a court to become a party to a case filed in the court based on an interest in the results of the case.

Negligence The failure to do something a reasonable person would do or doing something a reasonable person would not do.

Nominal damages A very small amount of money awarded to plaintiffs in cases in which there is no substantial injury. Nominal damages are awarded to recognize technical invasions of rights or breaches of duty or in cases where the injury is more substantial but the plaintiff fails to prove the amount.

Parens patriae Literally, "parent of the country." Refers to the role of each state as sovereign and guardian of persons under legal disability. This concept is the basis for activity by states to protect interests such as the health, comfort, and welfare of the people.

Per quod Literally, "whereby." A phrase used to designate facts concerning the consequences of defendant's actions on the plaintiff that serve as the basis for an award of special damages to the plaintiff.

Petition A formal, written request to a court asking the court to take certain action regarding a particular matter.

Physician-patient privilege The right of patients not to reveal or have revealed by their physicians the communications made between patients and physicians. The privilege is established in most states and therefore varies from state to state. The privilege belongs only to the patient and may be waived by the patient.

Plaintiff A person who sues in a civil case.

Pleading The formal, written statements by the parties to a suit of their respective claims and defenses.

Power of attorney A document authorizing another person to act on one's behalf. The other person is called the attorney in fact. The power of the attorney in fact is revoked on the death of the person who signed the power of attorney. The powers given to the attorney in fact may be general or for special purposes.

Prejudicial error Any error that substantially affects the legal rights and obligations of a party. A prejudicial error may result in a new trial and the reversal of a decision by the court.

Pretrial conference A meeting between opposing attorneys and the judge in a particular case. The purpose of the meeting is to define the key issues of the case, to secure stipulations, and to take all other steps necessary to aid in the disposition of the case. Such conferences are called at the discretion of the court. The decisions made at the conference are included in a written order that controls the future course of the case.

Pretrial discovery Any device used by parties before trial to obtain evidence for use at trial such as interrogatories, depositions, or requests for admission of facts.

Prima facie case Sufficient evidence presented by the plaintiff on which a decision that the plaintiff's claims are valid can reasonably be made.

Proximate cause The dominant cause or the cause producing injury. Any action producing injury, unbroken by any efficient intervening cause, and without which the injury would not have occurred.

Punitive damages Money awarded to the plaintiff over and above compensation for actual losses. Punitive damages are awarded in cases where the wrongdoing was aggravated by violence, oppression, malice, fraud, or wickedness. They are intended to compensate for mental anguish, shame, or degradation or to punish or make an example of the defendant.

Remand To send back. The sending back of a case by an appellate court to the court in which it was previously considered to have some further action taken on it.

Request for admissions Written statements of fact concerning a case that are submitted by the attorney for a party to a suit to the attorney for another party to the suit. The attorney who receives the request is required to either admit or deny each of the statements of fact submitted. Those statements that are admitted will be treated by the court as established and need not be proved at trial.

Res ipsa loquitur Literally, "the thing speaks for itself." Although the plaintiffs cannot testify to the exact cause of injury, they can prove (1) that the instrument causing injury was in defendants' exclusive control and (2) that the injury they sustained does not normally occur in the absence of negligence. Plaintiffs who prove both of these things can recover damages for negligence even though the exact circumstances of injury are known.

Res judicata A legal principle that says that once a *final* decision is made on a matter, the same question may not be raised at a later date.

Respondeat superior Literally, "let the master say." A basis for extending liability to include the employer for the wrongful acts of an employee. The doctrine is inapplicable where injury occurs when the employee is acting outside the legitimate scope of employment.

Retrial A new trial of a case that has already been tried at least once.

Stare decisis Literally, "to abide by or adhere to decided cases." The policy of courts in the United States to apply previously established principles of law to all future cases where the facts are substantially the same, even though the parties to the suit are not the same.

State action Activity of a state necessary to trigger the protection of the Fourteenth Amendment of the United States Constitution for private citizens.

Statute of limitations Legislative enactments establishing limits on the right to sue. Statutes of limitations declare that no one may sue unless the suit is filed within a specified period after the occurrence or injury that is the basis for the suit.

Stay A stopping by order of a court. A suspension of the case or some designated proceedings in it. A stay is a type of injunction with which a court freezes its proceedings at a particular point. It can be used to stop the case altogether or hold up only some phase of it.

Stipulation A voluntary agreement between opposing attorneys concerning disposition of a point that alleviates the need for proof of this point or for consideration, signed by the attorneys for all of the parties and placed on file as part of the court record.

Third-party defendant A party brought into a suit by the defendant who was not a party to the transaction on which the suit is based, but whose rights and liabilities may be affected by the suit.

Tort   A private or civil wrong or injury for which a court may award damages. Any civil suit except a suit for breach of contract. Three elements of every tort claim are (1) existence of a legal duty by the defendant to the plaintiff, (2) breach of this duty, *and* (3) resulting damage to the plaintiff.

Transcript   A word-for-word written record of a trial, hearing, or other proceeding.

Trial   An examination and determination of issues between the parties to a case by a court.

Trial by court or judge   A trial before a judge only, in contrast to a trial before a judge *and* jury.

Trial court   Judicial examination and determination of issues between the parties in a case.

Vicarious liability   Indirect legal responsibility.

Voir dire   Literally, "to speak the truth." Refers to the preliminary questioning that the court or attorneys conduct to determine the qualifications of a person to serve as a juror in a particular case.

Writ of certiorari   An order of an appellate court used when the court exercises discretion about whether or not to hear an appeal. If the writ is denied, the court refuses to hear the appeal, and the decision of the court that previously heard the case remains in effect. If the writ is granted, the appellate court will reconsider the case and perhaps change the decision of the lower court.

Writ of error   A writ issued from an appeals court to a trial court requiring the trial court to send the record of a case to the appeals court for reconsideration. The writ is based on errors of law apparent from the record. It is the beginning of a new suit to reverse a decision of a lower court and is not a continuation of any suit in a lower court.

Writ of habeas corpus   Literally, "you have the body." The primary function of this writ is to force the release of a person from unlawful imprisonment.

CHAPTER 9

Quality Assessment and Improvement

T. M. Marrelli

QUALITY: THE FOCUS OF THE NINETIES

The word *quality* has become omnipresent in health care and other business settings. Terms such as quality assurance (QA) have given way to the updated terms of total quality management (TQM), quality assessment and continuous quality improvement (QA/CQI), and total quality environment (TQE). It is important to note that QA is not unique to nursing or health care. Concepts about the provision of quality, in either products or services, have existed in the industrial and manufacturing realms for many years.

Quality processes, regardless of name, can be confusing to nurse managers and staff nurses involved in the daily integration of tracking and evaluating quality indicators. Quality in health care puts a value on meeting consumer needs in a safe and effective manner. This chapter includes an overview of the history leading to the heightened focus on quality in nursing practice in all health care settings.

WHY THE EMPHASIS ON QUALITY?

The reasons and pressures that contribute to the emphasis on quality are many and multifaceted. Regardless of the setting, the importance in health care of demonstrating quality will continue and intensify. The following are some of the main reasons why pressures to ensure quality have increased:

- Consumer awareness
- Cost-containment concerns
- Emphasis on effectiveness (doing more with less)
- Litigious society

- Trend towards a more service-oriented society
- Heightened awareness of human relation skills
- An objective way to quantify actions
- Opportunity for a competitive edge

QUALITY TODAY

As hospital quality improvement programs have evolved, patient outcomes are now recognized as valid indicators of quality of care. The marked increase in legal actions by consumers of health care services and products has contributed to the need for effective and ongoing quality programs. Clinical documentation becomes the written record demonstrating the nursing process and movement toward the achievement of patient-centered goals and objective outcomes. Nursing documentation often represents the quality of care provided. Unfortunately, if outcomes are not documented, the assumption can be made that the outcomes did not happen. Through complete documentation, the nurse can claim credit for meeting responsibilities inherent in the profession.

Documentation is also a vital adjunct to providing patient care. The new interdisciplinary team focus on quality assessment efforts creates an atmosphere for the entire health team to work together to achieve positive patient outcomes. Any effective QA/CQI program requires active participation by the nurse manager. Clinical documentation is the written evidence of this collaboration, which is evident in team meetings, conferences, and other activities. Because the clinical record is the only written source that chronicles a patient's stay, the importance of this record cannot be overemphasized. For that reason, a thorough discussion on documentation and the reasons for the emphasis on the quality of written communications is presented later in this chapter. This leads into a discussion on nursing standards of care. The documentation and nursing management–related standards of the JCAHO influence nursing practice in most settings; thus they have been included in the appendix of this chapter for your information.

DEFINING QUALITY

Nurses have been taught that quality care is present or occurs when patient needs are met in a manner satisfying to the patient and when the projected outcomes or goals are achieved. This includes physical, psychologic, emotional, and other needs related to the patient achieving the maximum potential functional independence on discharge. This all sounded clear, defined, and understandable when we were nursing neophytes. In practical terms it meant tracking patient falls or infections and doing retrospective chart audits on a regular basis to meet "quality requirements." In addition, the realm of QA activities historically fell to the nurse manager. For the nurse manager, it is important to know that quality comes from people doing effective work daily. As managers, we know the only way to accomplish work is through staff members. With this in mind, the key is empowering the staff and building teams to accomplish consistent quality outcomes. Environments that have clear organizational goals and communicate these with the staff, act on them daily as role models, and nurture and reward staff excellence are working toward quality. The attitude that CQI is an ongoing, dynamic process is expected and welcomed in settings where staff and managers integrate quality in daily practice.

THE IMPORTANCE OF NURSING QUALITY PROGRAMS

Today, the quality process demands participation from nurses rendering care. Quality programs may be decentralized, with ties to the overall institution's quality programs. Quality affects every person and facet of health care provided. This encompasses the admitting clerk, housekeeping, and volunteer services and includes the myriad people interacting with patients and their families or caregivers daily. Nursing is a major component of any health care setting and the foundation of the institution's overall quality program. Because nursing affects patient care services directly and historically has had input into the actual quality of care received, nursing is recognized as the leader in quality activities in most health settings. To clarify the numerous terms and phrases that are all a part of QA/CQI, lists in this chapter of such terms are alphabetically organized with explanations of the process or term listed and commonly used when discussing or implementing QA or CQI programs. Where possible, examples have been included.

Deming's Definition of Quality

Defining what quality means, in today's complex practice settings, with increased consumerism, decreased lengths of stay, and myriad other factors, is a difficult task. There are numerous definitions in the current environment. Deming's definition of quality is, "Delivering what the consumer wants, the first time and everytime, . . . a product or a service [that] both meets the consumer's needs and is free of defects."[1]

The simplicity of this definition may obscure the actual difficulty of achieving patient/client goals when numerous factors, technologies, and caregivers are involved. We know what "quality" looks like; a patient with positive outcomes. To be truly effective, quality goals must cut across all organizational lines and boundaries. The health care team must function as one unit, with the organization's goals clearly in mind. Finally, staff demonstrations of quality must be effectively reinforced through rewards.

Certain words or phrases are unique to quality. These terms are being updated very rapidly, and use can vary in different health settings. The following are the hallmarks.

12 FREQUENTLY HEARD QUALITY PHRASES

✔ **Chart audits**—Historically, chart audits were what nursing units relied on as the major, if not only, QA yardstick. The words *quality assurance* themselves have given way to the new terms *quality improvement* or, simply, quality. In the past, these chart audits tended to be administratively focused reviews. Now they are more clinically focused as quality moves toward a patient-outcome orientation. Chart audits are an objective, demonstrable "trail" that can objectively measure QI using a quantifiable process. Examples include (1) a completed nursing discharge summary on each patient's record for a specified date and (2) that all patients signed a patient's bill of rights within 4 hours of admission.

✔ **Demonstrating quality**—QA/QI should be demonstrated using objective findings. The most common example is a written clinical entry in the medical record.

✔ **Quality indicators**—Indicators are the specific processes or entities to be evaluated. These are usually measurable and objective. An example is a patient's knowledge on discharge, including the drawing up and administration of subcutaneous insulin, emergency measures, and use of a glucometer. This knowledge was evidenced by the documentation in the record that recorded the patient's actions and verbalization before discharge.

✔ **Quality assessment**—QA is the evaluation phase of the measuring of clinical or objective indicators. These findings or results are evaluated to ascertain the need for change or modification in practice or care provided.

✔ **Quality circles**—Such a circle is the method of achieving work products or goals by the use of effective teams. Though used historically in production environments, quality circles are being seen in all types of environments, including services. Quality circles usually involve a group of team members given a specific work task.

✔ **Quality improvement**—QI is an effort characterized by the need for and identification of opportunity for continual improvement. It usually involves team processes, structured and effective recognition of excellence, and established, attainable goals. It is usually integrated into the TQE program of the organization. It has become more ongoing in the newer term *continuous quality improvement (CQI)*.

✔ **Total quality management**—TQM is a business practice that is employee-centered and consumer-oriented and consumer-controlled and that emphasizes continual efforts toward product or service improvement. TQM is characterized by clear, ongoing, open communications; effective teamwork; total organizational commitment to common goals; and open employee involvement on a daily basis.

✔ **Quality standards**—A quality standard is a designated level of care that must be maintained in professional nursing practice for that practice to be considered acceptable. In nursing practice, these are usually referred to as standards of care.

✔ **Structural QA/QI**—Any condition that is conducive to providing quality of care is a structural QA/QI. An example could be an ongoing hospital QA committee or a policy that all patients receive a patient satisfaction survey within 30 days of discharge.

✔ **Total quality environment (TQE)**—TQE is the updated and improved term in some settings for TQM. This phrase obviously connotes that quality is respected and supported at all levels of any hierarchy. Some consider it to be more encompassing and, as such, more successful in achieving QA/QI.

✔ **Total quality management (TQM)**—TQM stresses belief in the importance and contribution of all team workers to the achievement of organizational goals in an environment that supports quality. Ongoing team member and staff training, rewards, and clearly defined organizational goals are the hallmarks of successful TQM. In addition, appreciating all employees, regardless of organizational chart position, contributes to effective teams and participatory management styles.

✔ **Unit-based QA/CQI**—Hospitals and other health organizations or units continue to streamline for increased productivity. This change brings the workers closer to the problems and simultaneously respects their input into effective solutions. Decentralization will continue, and it is thought that this trend will result in small teams or "clusters" that self-manage with clear organizational goals and minimal input from management. Unit-based QA/CQI allows nurse managers to focus on problems and develop unique solutions to the problems that work for their special environment.

The Emphasis on Quality and Consumerism in Health Care

As patients become more effective consumers of health care, their knowledge level and expectation for quality care increases. Because nursing practice involves many decisions, the responsibility for and the accountability to the consumer also increases. An effective quality program evaluates the health setting standards of patient care and the nursing standards of practice. Nurses are in the key, multifaceted role that affects patients, being the predominant health provider. Many health care programs have patients complete a survey about the care they received. These patient satisfaction surveys are useful in identifying problems and trends perceived by patients regarding the care they received. Nurse managers should share this information with the staff, to improve care where needed and to compliment staff on a continued job well done. These written evaluations of the care provided can provide a wealth of knowledge to the nurse manager. Sometimes these surveys are done by other services in the hospital. For example, the public relations department may have the responsibility for the creation, distribution, retrieval, and data analysis of the patient satisfaction surveys. The nurse manager may have to work with the public relations staff or the nursing executive to receive feedback on a particular unit. Again, the effective nurse manager may then communicate the findings to the staff and work with them to designate action items for implementation to continue ensuring quality.

MORE QUALITY TERMS

✔ **ANA**—The American Nurse's Association is an example of a professional organization that creates and distributes standards developed by those with expertise in a chosen area of practice. These standards are then published and shared with nursing colleagues. Standards are one of the vital components of a profession. Belonging to professional nursing organizations contributes to quality outcomes.

✔ **Committees (quality)**—Committees are the formal structure created to communicate QA/QI processes that occur on an ongoing basis. The minutes of these meetings are the objective source of identified problems, corrective action plans, implementation, new findings, reevaluations of the problems, and the resolution of identified problems. The committee usually has a goal statement, which may include the formal membership roster, the committee objectives, and a description of the reporting mechanism that integrates the QA/QI programs into the total organizational quality programs. Committees often have process standards, specific member functions, and regularly scheduled meeting times.

DOCUMENTATION

Webster's New World Dictionary[2] defines documentation as "the supplying of documentary evidence . . . and the collecting, abstracting, and coding of printed or written information for future reference." This simple definition fits all of the varied and important roles that documentation, or the process of documenting and demonstrating delivery of patient care, assumes in health care. Nursing entries that appear in the medical record reflect the standard of nursing care, as well as the specific care provided to the patient. Other health care team members make decisions for further care based on the nursing entries. And today, numerous third-party payors make legal and quality judgements, as well as administrative and payment decisions, based on the medical record. Nurses have many responsibilities, all ultimately directed toward patient care. Because of these responsibilities, the actual task of documentation must sometimes be relegated to the end of the shift.

According to the AHA, patient charts now average 70 to 100 pages. This means that most midsized hospitals process 250,000 to 360,000 pieces of medical information each year.[3] The typical medical record may be read by a minimum of 10 persons during a patient's initial 24 hours in a health facility. These may include the admitting or attending physician, three nurses on different shifts, the utilization review specialist, several nurse aides, and a dietician. They may also include a surgeon, an anesthesiologist, and various technicians and therapists. With so many people depending on the medical record as a reliable and up-to-date source of patient information, the importance of the data contained in the record becomes evident.

THE PROFESSIONAL NURSE'S ROLE IN DOCUMENTATION

The professional nurse's entries in the patient's clinical record are recognized as a significant contribution documenting the standard of care provided to a patient. As the practice of nursing has become more complex, so too have the factors that influence the purposes of documentation. These factors include the requirements of regulatory agencies, health insurance payors, accreditation organizations, consumers of health care, and legal entities. The nurse must try to satisfy these various requirements, all at once, often with precious few moments in which to accomplish this important task.

Any nurse writing a clinical entry today could be trying simultaneously to meet the standards of JCAHO, various insurers, state and federal laws and regulations, and other professional organizations. Fortunately, most hospitals have integrated many of these requirements, when possible, into hospital policy or procedure manuals.

The written clinical record is the professional nurse's best defense against litigation when malpractice or negligence is alleged. The increased specialization of health care providers and the complexity of patient problems and associated technology have contributed to multiple and varied services being provided to patients in a shortened time frame. The medical record is the only source of written communication, and sometimes the only source of any communication, for all team members. The members not only contribute their individual assessments of interventions and outcomes, but actually base their subsequent actions on the record of events provided by other team members. As such, the actual entries must be recorded as soon as possible after a change in the patient's condition is noted, an intervention occurs, or the response to a treatment is observed. Nurses can have their practice well represented and quality demonstrated through thorough, effective documentation.

FUNCTION OF THE MEDICAL RECORD

Clear documentation in the medical record is highly important because this record is:

- The only written source that chronicles a patient's stay from admission through discharge.
- The primary source for reference and communication among members of the health care team.
- The only documentation that supports insurance coverage (payment) or denial.
- The only evidence of the basis on which patient care decisions were made.
- The only legal record.
- The foundation for evaluation of the care provided.
- The basis for staff education or other study.
- The objective source for the facility's licensing and accreditation review (e.g., JCAHO, the American Osteopathic Association Standards).

The above factors have contributed to an environment in which the nurse has increased responsibilities for documentation and a shortened time frame for producing such documentation because of the decrease in patient lengths of stay. This written record is the only account of a patient's stay. Many QA/QI processes involve the medical record for these reasons.

KEY TERMS RELATED TO DOCUMENTATION

✔ **Outcome criteria**—Outcome criteria are the desired results on completion or the objective (or demonstrable) evidence observed at the end of care (e.g., a patient's anticipated knowledge or activity level on discharge). In a specific case, a patient with diabetes mellitus returned to self-care status. Patient able to demonstrate all activities noted on the diabetes mellitus checklist on discharge and patient verbalized that initial complaints were resolved and needs met.

✔ **Process**—A process is specifically how the care is provided. An example would be a standard that requires that all patients receive a complete assessment within so many (specify) hours of admission. The specific parameters that must be included in the assessment would also be identified.

✔ **Standards of care**—There is a growing emphasis on the standardization of care, policies, and procedures. All patients or clients are entitled to a certain level, or standard, of care. As patients become more proactive consumers in the purchase of needed health care services, patient satisfaction with care provided becomes the key to the facility's reputation and ultimate survival. Nurses, because of their healing skills and other areas of proficiency, are pivotal in fostering patient satisfaction. The roles of the nurse as patient advocate, listener, and teacher have become widely accepted in recent years. With these roles comes the responsibility of maintaining the hallmarks of any profession. These include licensure, education, certification or other credentialing processes, and other, ongoing educational requirements. Standards of care in nursing today are varied and include nursing specialty association standards and ANA national, state, and local standards that define the acceptable level of practice. These standards are vital to the professional nurse's ongoing education. For this reason, it is important that the nurse remain informed on all areas of practice that affect the provision of care.

TIPS FOR IMPLEMENTING QUALITY PROGRAMS

An effective quality program has many facets. The following are examples that may help you ensure quality on your unit or in your program.

✔ Communicate clear definitions of the responsibilities for the quality program.

✔ Choose indicators your nursing staff identify.

✔ Make the indicators objective.

✔ Provide comprehensive orientation to all new staff members.

✔ Generally, match the skills of the staff with the needs of the patient.

✔ Focus on the process, not the staff member.

✔ Create an environment where staff members are encouraged to identify problems early.

✔ Provide appropriate and ongoing in-service education for staff members.

✔ Actively participate in assessing the quality of care provided.

✔ Read and use any reports available to you that help identify trends (e.g., infection control reports or antibiotic use control sheet).

✔ Involve the entire interdisciplinary team, where possible.

✔ Develop a routine to automatically and objectively review a minimum number of patient charts weekly. Provide timely and specific feedback to staff members.

✔ Implement a nurse peer professional review of the documentation.

✔ Keep lines of communication open at all levels. Talk to patients, their families, and friends about what you can do better.

✔ Read the patient satisfaction surveys that are returned. Implement the changes recommended. If your program does not currently do this, begin a program. Involve public relations, your nursing staff, and patients in developing the tool to be used.

✔ Consider what you would want as a consumer of services.

✔ Be open and listen to new ideas from any source on how to achieve quality.

✔ Monitor that needs of patients are met on discharge.

✔ Value "guest relations." Train your staff to be empathetic with all patients, peers, and visitors and to respect their unique fears and needs.

✔ Ask your staff about ways to improve patient care and more effective ways of doing tasks on your unit. Implement an "idea box" and hold brainstorming sessions on quality.

✔ Volunteer to be a nursing representative on the nursing quality council and the hospital- or agency-wide council.

✔ Reward behaviors that support these goals.

SUMMARY

Quality will continue to be the focus of health care in years to come. Consumer-driven health care has focused attention on patient/client rights, spiraling health care costs, and increased accountability by providers of health care for an effective quality product. These multifaceted pressures from various sources can be stressful. For these reasons, quality must be pervasive in all activities at all levels. It can encompass any factor that can be objectively assessed or outcome evaluated. All problems or trends can be filtered through the QA/QI processes. Many leaders in quality management believe that increased productivity, results, and financial viability come with effectively managed quality programs. The nurse manager, as role model and team leader, is the key to a successful, functional, and result-oriented quality program.

REFERENCES

1. Curtain L, Zurlage C: Cornerstones of healthcare in the nineties: forging a framework of excellence—a report on a landmark conference, *Nurs Manage* 22(4):32-43, 1991.
2. Guralnik DB, editor-in-chief: *Webster's new world dictionary*, ed 2, college, 1982, Simon & Schuster.
3. American Hospital Association: Medical records: increasing importance, heavier workload. In *Side-by-side profiles*, Chicago, 1990, The AHA. pp 1-4.

JCAHO Standards For Nursing Management Functions

JCAHO is a professional body that creates and measures standards. Facilities or health organizations pay JCAHO professional surveyors to evaluate their services, setting, or program objectively. The awarding of the JCAHO accreditation is an indicator of a high level of care (quality) demonstrated at the health setting. JCAHO evaluations are in-depth and include staff, patient, and family interviews. For convenience, the standards directly related to the nursing management functions are included in this appendix.

NC.3 The nurse executive and other appropriate registered nurses develop hospital-wide patient care programs, policies, and procedures that describe how the nursing care needs of patients or patient populations are assessed, evaluated, and met.

> **NC.3.1** Policies and procedures, based on nursing standards of patient care and standards of nursing practice, describe and guide the nursing care provided.
>
> > **NC.3.1.1** The nurse executive has the authority and responsibility for establishing standards of nursing practice.
> >
> > **NC.3.1.2** The policies, procedures, nursing standards of patient care, and standards of nursing practice are
> >
> > > **NC.3.1.2.1** developed by the nurse executive, registered nurses, and other designated nursing staff members
> > >
> > > **NC.3.1.2.2** defined in writing
> > >
> > > **NC.3.1.2.3** approved by the nurse executive or a designee(s)

206

NC.3.1.2.4 used, as indicated, in the assessment of the quality of patient care

NC.3.1.3 Review of policies and procedures include information about the relevance of policies, procedures, nursing standards of patient care, and standards of nursing practice in actual use; ethical and legal concerns; current scientific knowledge; and findings from quality assessment and improvement activities and other evaluation mechanisms, as appropriate.

NC.3.2 Nursing staff members have a defined mechanism for addressing ethical issues in patient care.

NC.3.2.1 When the hospital has an ethics committee or other defined structures for addressing ethical issues in patient care, nursing staff members participate.

NC.3.3 Policies and procedures are developed in collaboration with other clinical and administrative groups, when appropriate.

NC.3.3.1 The nurse executive, or a designee(s), participates in the hospital admissions system to coordinate patient requirements for nursing care with available nursing resources.

NC.3.3.1.1 In making the decision when or where to admit and/or transfer a patient, consideration is given to the ability of the nursing staff to assess and meet the patient's nursing care needs.

NC.3.4 Policies and procedures describe the mechanism used to assign nursing staff members to meet patient care needs.

NC.3.4.1 There are sufficient qualified nursing staff members to meet the nursing care needs of patients throughout the hospital.

NC.3.4.1.1 The criteria for employment, deployment, and assignment of nursing staff members are approved by the nurse executive.

NC.3.4.2 Nurse staffing plans for each unit define the number and mix of nursing personnel in accordance with current patient care needs.

NC.3.4.2.1 In designing and assessing nurse staffing plans, the hospital gives appropriate consideration to the utilization of registered nurses, licensed practical/vocational nurses, nursing assistants, and other nursing personnel and to the potential contribution these personnel can make to the delivery of efficient and effective patient care.

NC.3.4.2.2 The staffing schedules are reviewed and adjusted as necessary to meet defined patient needs and unusual occurrences.

NC.3.4.2.3 Appropriate and sufficient support services are available to allow nursing staff members to meet the nursing care needs of patients and their significant other(s).

NC.3.4.2.4 Staffing levels are adequate to support participation of nursing staff members, as assigned, in committees/meetings and in educational and quality assessment and improvement activities.

NC.5 The nurse executive and other nursing leaders participate with leaders from the governing body, management, medical staff, and clinical areas in the hospital's decision-making structures and processes.

NC. 5.1 Nursing services are directed by a nurse executive who is a registered nurse qualified by advanced education and management experience.

NC.5.1.1 If the hospital utilizes a decentralized organizational structure, there is an identified nurse leader at the executive level to provide authority and accountability for, and coordination of, the nurse executive functions.

NC.5.1.2 When the hospital is part of a multihospital system, there is a mechanism(s) for the hospital's nurse executive to participate in policy decisions affecting patient care services at relevant levels of corporate decision making within the system.

NC.5.1.2.1 The mechanism(s) is used to enhance the exchange of information about, as well as participation in, improving the nursing care provided to patients in the hospital.

NC.5.1.2.2 The mechanism(s) is defined in writing.

NC.5.2 The nurse executive or a designee(s) participates with leaders from the governing body, management, medical staff, and clinical areas in developing the hospital's mission, strategic plans, budgets, resource allocation, operation plans, and policies.

NC.5.2.1 The nurse executive develops the nursing budget in collaboration with other nursing leaders and other hospital personnel.

NC.5.2.2 The nurse executive and other nursing leaders participate in the ongoing review of the hospital's mission, strategic plans, and policies.

NC.5.3 The nurse executive and other nursing leaders participate with leaders from the governing body, management, medical staff, and clinical areas in planning, promoting, and conducting hospitalwide quality monitoring and improvement activities.

NC.5.3.1 Registered nurses evaluate current nursing practice and patient care delivery models to improve the quality and efficiency of patient care.

NC.5.3.2 The nurse executive and other nursing leaders participate in developing and implementing mechanisms for collaboration between nursing staff members, physicians, and other clinical practitioners.

NC.5.4 The nurse executive and other nursing leaders are responsible for developing, implementing, and evaluating programs to promote the recruitment, retention, development, and continuing education of nursing staff members.

NC.5.4.1 The nurse executive and other nursing leaders participate in developing and implementing mechanisms for recognizing the expertise and performance of nursing staff members engaged in patient care.

NC.5.4.2 The nurse executive and other nursing leaders collaborate with governing body and other management and clinical leaders to develop mechanisms for promoting the educational and advancement goals of hospital staff members.

NC.5.5 The nurse executive or a designee(s) participates in evaluating, selecting, and integrating health care technology and information management systems that support patient care needs and the efficient utilization of nursing resources.

NC.5.5.1 The use of efficient interactive information management systems for nursing, other clinical (e.g., dietary, pharmacy, physical therapy), and nonclinical information is facilitated wherever appropriate.

NC.5.6 When the hospital provides clinical facilities for nursing education programs, appropriate nursing leaders collaborate with nursing educators to influence curricula, including clinical and/or managerial learning experiences.

Reprinted with permission from *Accreditation manual for hospitals,* 1992 ed, Oakbrook Terrace, Ill, 1991, Joint Commission on Accreditation of Healthcare Organizations.

Taking Care of Yourself and Your Staff

Patricia M. Feeney

MAINTAINING BALANCE UNDER STRESS

Nicholson, a registered nurse and certified Stress Management Program Director through the American Institute of Preventive Medicine, proposed a definition of stress as it applies to the nursing profession. After reviewing the work of Hans Selye and many others, Nicholson suggested that stress in nursing is

. . . a phenomenon that is characterized by a response to a certain occurrence. This response may be interpreted as positive or negative by the individual and can affect biologic processes, which may result eventually in wear or tear on one's physical, psychologic, behavioral, and/or emotional well-being.[1]

Stress in the Nursing Profession

Careers in nursing and nursing management bring with them careers in managing stress. As a nurse and nurse manager, it is important to your personal and professional long-term success to integrate stress management skills into your life.

A critical element in managing stress in the nursing profession is accepting that stress does and always will exist. Some of these stresses are unique to our profession. Foxall and others[2] compared the frequency and sources of nursing job stress perceived by intensive care, hospice, and medical-surgical nurses. Although the groups assigned different degrees of stress to various aspects of their work, the overall frequency of job stress was similar among the three groups.

Numerous studies detail the sources of stress experienced by nurses. Although many of these stresses may be identified in non-health care settings, many stresses found in the nursing profession

211

are products of the environment. Examples include dying patients, cardiac arrests, communicable disease, and upset families.

Stresses in the nursing workplace that also are identified in non-health care settings, such as increased workload and conflicts with staff members, can be intensified in the health care setting. These common or universal job stresses affect nurses more because they directly affect patient care.

Nurse Managers: A Two-Fold Responsibility

As a nurse manager, you accept a two-fold responsibility in stress management: (1) guiding and supporting your staff as they experience stress, and (2) coping with stress as it affects you. Although these responsibilities seem self-evident, many managers are not successful in supporting their staff, themselves, or both. Sadly, a failure to support one or the other generally results in a failure to support both.

For example, if your concern rests primarily with your own stress and coping mechanisms, your staff will recognize this fact. Eventually, they will resent your lack of support and may begin to experience excessive stress themselves. Over time, these feelings may result in high staff turnover, decreased staff performance, and unhappy patients and physicians. These factors in turn lead to excessive stress for you.

Conversely, if your concern is exclusively for your staff, eventually you will become emotionally drained, resentful, and overly stressed. As these feelings take their toll on your well-being, your ability to manage and support your staff will diminish. This diminishing performance in turn will lead to excessive stress for your staff.

It is imperative that you understand the importance of attending to the needs of your staff, as well as to your own needs—consistently and simultaneously.

Stress Evaluation Exercises: Introduction

This chapter contains stress evaluation exercises. These exercises are designed to help you identify and evaluate stress in your work environment. The exercises include stress self-knowledge, stress coping mechanisms, and signs of unmanaged stress. You may use these exercises alone or in brainstorming sessions with your peers. The exercises may also be used in staff support groups that are conducted by a professional facilitator.

The stress evaluation exercises are tools to help you identify stress and their accompanying problems. In most cases, you and your staff will be able to respond to stress effectively. However, you may find that you, an individual on your staff, or your staff as a group is experiencing stress beyond normal levels or is developing a serious problem in response to stress. If so, seek professional support for yourself and/or the employees experiencing the problem. Please refer to the section, "When You Identify A Serious Staff Problem" of this chapter for further discussion.

SOURCES OF STRESS IN THE NURSING ENVIRONMENT

Once you are committed to monitoring and managing stress in the work place, a clear understanding of the sources of stress is critical. Undoubtedly, you have a good sense of the types of events or situations that create stress for you. Most nurse managers have spent a considerable part of their career in staff level positions and are well acquainted with the rigors of the profession.

It is important to note that the areas of stress which affect you may not be the same as those which most affect the members of your staff. For example, off-shift scheduling affects people differently and may affect them differently at various points in their lives. Working the night shift profoundly affects some people's sense of emotional equilibrium and their sleep patterns. Yet, some nurses enjoy an occasional rotation to nights and some happily choose to work nights full-time.

Caring for dying patients is stressful. Yet for some nurses, caring for a dying patient is not experienced as a negative stress. These nurses may exercise hidden strengths and qualities and be deeply satisfied by the experience. For other nurses, caring for a dying patient may be deeply depressing.

It is helpful to review an inventory of the sources of stress in the nursing work place so that you can be sensitive to the differences among your staff members and guard against generalizing your experiences to them.

Lees and Ellis investigated a variety of common stresses in their study[3] of nursing staff, nursing students, and students who left nurse training. The following are the stresses they identified, with the stresses most frequently cited appearing at the top of the list.

COMMONLY OCCURRING STRESSES[3]

✔ Understaffing

✔ Dealing with death and dying

✔ Conflict with nurses

✔ Overwork

✔ Conflict with doctors

✔ Hours

✔ Cardiac arrests

✔ Responsibility/accountability

✔ Training junior staff

✔ Dealing with relatives

✔ Lack of resources (beds/equipment)

✔ Aggressive patients

✔ Study/exams

✔ Carrying out certain nursing procedures

✔ Feeling inadequate to carry out procedures

✔ Seeing patients in distress

✔ Staff rough with patients

✔ Conflict with others (administrators, dietitians)

✔ Child abuse

✔ Dealing with overdose patients

✔ Living in nurses' home

✔ Open visiting

✔ Working off-shifts

✔ Disorganization of workloads

✔ Being in a new situation for the first time

✔ Heat in the hospital

Simms and others investigated some of these same stresses in their study[4] of nursing burnout. The following is a list of the exhausting activities cited by nurses in their study. The activities at the top of the list are those most frequently cited.

EXHAUSTING ACTIVITIES [4]

✔ Decreased staffing

✔ Negativism on part of staff

✔ Demanding families

✔ No time for breaks or lunches

✔ Increased patient load

✔ Too many patients

✔ Dealing with difficult people

✔ Being on their feet all day

✔ Routine patient care

✔ Transferring patients in beds

✔ Mandatory overtime

✔ Running errands

✔ Problems with other departments

✔ Dealing with staff conflict

✔ Patients and families unwilling to accept diagnosis

✔ Patients who are self-abusing

✔ Paperwork

✔ Cardiac arrests

✔ Caring for debilitated patients

✔ Meetings in other buildings

✔ Not being busy

✔ Being on call

✔ Orienting new staff

✔ Repetitive teaching

✔ Scheduling and staffing

✔ Responding to alarms

✔ Trying to alleviate patients' pain

Nurses may experience additional stresses when they care for patients with specialized needs or with an illness such as AIDS or hepatitis, which can be threatening to one's own health. Although caring for a patient with a communicable disease may cause anxiety for nurses, there are several other, less visible, special-care situations that may concern nurses.

Some of these situations are those which pose a real or imagined threat to the health of the nurse or the nurse's family. For example, nursing personnel in neonatal intensive care units are frequently called on to hold or otherwise manage infants during x-ray procedures. If the infant is in isolation, does the nurse contaminate a lead apron (creating the need for time-consuming decontamination), put on and cover the apron, or simply hold the infant without protecting herself from the radiation? This kind of decision, invariably made in a split second, may create stress for the nurse making the decision.

Nurses on oncology units regularly manage chemotherapy agents and waste products of patients receiving these agents. The threat of possible exposure to mutagenic chemicals may bring considerable stress to the nurses managing these patients. Nurses who plan to have children, particularly those who are pregnant or actively trying to become pregnant or father a child, may experience additional stress in care settings where they may be exposed to mutagenic chemotherapy agents, communicable diseases, radiation, and other threats to their ability to bear or father a healthy child.

In addition to the stresses intrinsic to the workplace, nurses, like all people, may experience personal problems that magnify the stress at work.

STRESS EVALUATION EXERCISE: STRESS SELF-KNOWLEDGE

Develop a list of all possible sources of stress in your workplace. Recognize that there are no "rights" or "wrongs" in your evaluation and that not every stress identified will apply directly to you or to every nurse on your staff. The purpose of your evaluation is simply to identify sources of stress, not to assign blame for the stress or to provide solutions.

By limiting the first task at hand to a simple process of identification, the pressure to solve—or deny—problems is eliminated.

STRESSES FOR NURSE MANAGERS

The nurse manager is vulnerable to stresses that are inherent to the two-fold role of nurse and manager.

One source of stress is a result of the nurse manager's position in the organization. New managers typically are first-line supervisors and must report to a supervisor above them. In fact, there may be several layers of personnel between the nurse manager and top management. This "layering" of management can be a significant source of stress.

For example, when you receive top management's communications through your supervisor, he or she may alter the positioning or emphasis of the communication to motivate you to act positively. This is not necessarily a problem. In fact, you will find yourself doing the same in your communications with your staff. As you become an effective manager who is more acquainted with the staff, you will learn how to report information so that the staff understands the content and is motivated to take positive action.

However, this filtering of information can become a problem for you when your supervisor, committed to his or her own agenda, misinterprets information and communicates misinterpretations to you. You then receive communication that is inconsistent with top management's message and possibly inconsistent with the organization's objectives. You, in turn, communicate this misinformation to your staff, who ultimately may experience their own stress related to this situation.

OTHER SOURCES OF STRESS FOR THE NURSE MANAGER

✔ Feeling "sandwiched" between your staff and your supervisor.

✔ Being responsible for patient care/client services delivered by each member of your staff.

✔ Accepting fiscal responsibility for your area of supervision.

✔ Being responsible for staff turnover in your area of supervision.

✔ Serving as liaison in physician-nurse relationships.

✔ Serving as liaison in staff-upper management relationships.

✔ Having responsibility for staff education and training.

✔ Handling conflicts with role expectations from your staff and your supervisor.

✔ Handling internal role conflicts concerning your responsibilities as a nurse and as a manager.

✔ Scheduling staffing for your area of supervision.

✔ Making unpopular decisions.

✔ Facilitating communications between your staff and upper management.

✔ Evaluating staff.

✔ Setting reasonable, objective goals for your staff.

✔ Taking disciplinary action against a staff member.

✔ Terminating a staff member.

✔ Hiring a staff member.

✔ Responding constructively to unmanaged stress among your staff.

✔ Recognizing the signs of unmanaged stress among your staff.

✔ Recognizing signs and symptoms of unmanaged stress within yourself.

✔ Facilitating open communication among your staff with each other and with you.

✔ Conducting staff meetings.

✔ Accepting criticism from your supervisor and from your staff.

✔ Taking a vacation from your job.

✔ Learning to delegate appropriately.

✔ Being seen as the "bad guy" by your staff.

✔ Being regarded as "omnipotent" by your staff.

✔ Having little orientation for your management role.

✔ Dealing with employees who merely want a "job," and are not committed to their profession or career.

✔ Keeping a balance at work when your personal problems seem to be following you to work.

✔ Managing an employee who brings her or his personal problems to work.

✔ Other stresses you have identified.

Managing an employee with a personal problem warrants a brief discussion. Employees' personal problems are just that—*their* personal problems. Nonetheless, if one of your employees is experiencing difficulty in her or his personal life, be it financial, marital, child-related, or so forth, it is not uncommon for the employee to bring the problem to work. Sometimes an employee may be so stressed and distracted by personal concerns that her or his job performance is affected. Although you must address the employee's performance deficits, it is especially important in these circumstances to do so with compassion.

If an employee confides a personal problem to you, it will be important to keep a balance between showing concern and caring, and trying to correct the problem. Keep in mind that you are not a therapist and are not equipped to psychologically counsel your staff. You cannot remedy your staff's personal problems. Sometimes the greatest support you can offer is to suggest that the employee seek guidance from a community resource or trained professional. Examples of resources are discussed in the section, "When You Identify a Serious Staff Problem."

You have probably become acquainted with many of the sources of stress on the nurse manager's stress list. It may also be helpful to brainstorm sources of stress with your peer group. Discussing sources of stress with other first-line managers can help validate your perceptions. This process also can strengthen your peer relationships.

THE MANAGER-STAFF RELATIONSHIP

To understand the stress you experience as a nurse manager, it is helpful to examine the nature of your relationships with your staff and with your supervisor.

A guiding principle behind successfully managing your staff is a clear understanding of the psychology at work. As simplistic as this sounds, this psychology often is neglected when a nurse manager is caught up in day-to-day operational management responsibilities.

How the Staff Views the Manager

Regardless of your age, experience, and education, generally your staff will view you as an authority figure. This authority is vested in you because you have a supervisory job title.

Your staff will expect you to respond to their needs, alleviate the stress of their job, and guide them through troubled times. Over time, the authority your staff vests in you must be proven, or the staff will lose the respect for you that is important to successful manager-staff relationships. Nonetheless, knowing that you arrive on the job with a certain measure of authority can boost your confidence as you face the challenges ahead.

But what does this authority mean? At first glance, it seems great. People will listen when you speak. People will work harder and do their best if they believe you are aware of their performance. You have at your disposal several ways to motivate your staff: pats on the back, performance reviews, certificates of merit, continuing education days, and other perks you can provide.

However, your position of authority brings with it some other, less desirable, effects. People will listen when you speak, but they may criticize you for what you say, regardless of whether the blame is accurately assigned. For example, if you have to report staff cutbacks that have been formulated by upper management, *you* may be blamed for the cutbacks. If you correct someone's nursing technique, you may be considered "too hard," "unrealistic," or "out of touch with the real world."

Staff cutbacks and correcting a nurse's technique may be necessary, but they will still create stress for you and your staff. As the manager, you must be aware of this inherent stress so that you communicate with your staff in a positive way, without placing undue stress on them or on yourself.

Open Communication

Effective communication as a nurse manager is not measured by how much your staff likes you. Rather, it is measured by how well you relate verbally and nonverbally in a clear, respectful manner, listening to your staff, encouraging comments and constructive criticism, and creating an environment in which each individual's opinions are respected. As the manager, you ultimately must make decisions on matters related to personnel and operations in your area of responsibility. These decisions—though not always popular—must be respected.

A manager who has created an environment of open communication may experience what appears to be a lack of support in the face of an unpopular decision. Staff members who feel comfortable expressing disagreement and concerns will be more apt to criticize—and sometimes to do so unfairly. It will be important to remember that the staff is simply expressing openly what they would think covertly in a less communicative environment. Even if you are unable or unwilling to alter your decision, listening attentively to your staff's dissatisfaction will provide a degree of relief from the stress brought on by your decision.

Do not underestimate your staff and expect that unpopular decisions will necessarily make you unpopular. Sometimes a manager finds unexpected support in the face of a tough decision. This support may not be apparent until the staff has had the opportunity to assimilate the decision. In most cases, your staff will recognize a fair or necessary decision for what it is and respect you for making it.

Regardless of your staff's response to an unpopular decision, you must bear in mind your first priority: to live up to your job responsibilities to the best of your abilities. This generally means doing what is best for the patients/clients first, and then for your staff.

Balancing Your Emotional Needs and Your Job Responsibilities

Because your job can be draining, take care to see that your emotional needs are met in constructive ways. Avoid using your staff as the key source of your emotional support. This does not mean you must tense up if one of your staff extends a helping hand or offers a kind or caring remark. (This would be wonderful!) However, keep in perspective how much you can expect of your staff. Although you may come to enjoy being with and care about many of the staff members, relying on them to support you emotionally is not fair. If you become dependent on one or more of your staff members for support, your judgment will be clouded and it will be difficult for you to do your job.

Although most nurse managers want their staffs to like and care about them, focusing on this desire can create serious problems. Most experienced nurse managers know that it is difficult to do a good job *and* be liked all of the time. Some nurse managers—just like some of the population at large—have a strong emotional need to be liked. If this is true of you, it is important that you continually assess your performance to be sure you are doing your job, not running for office. In fact, even experienced managers may be vulnerable to the desire to "run for office" when things seem particularly tough in running their department, clinic, or home health agency.

Conversely, some managers, in an attempt to establish their authority, tend to go overboard and create an environment akin to a police state. This pitfall, as well as "running for office," seems particularly common with first-time managers and is an understandable mistake. It's difficult to gauge how to present oneself, or how strong to come on with the staff, when the nurse manager has had no previous management experience.

Inventory of Your Management Practices

You may want to take a mental inventory of your management practices. The following are questions designed as triggers to help you evaluate your behavior and to build a healthy work environment—an environment in which your staff feels able to communicate with you and contribute to decision-making, but is respectful of your responsibilities as a manager. The questions also will help you measure your management "comfort level" (i.e., how well you are accepting the nurse manager's responsibilities). Following the questions are guidelines to evaluate your responses.

MANAGEMENT PRACTICES—QUESTIONS TO ASK YOURSELF

✔ Before I report a management decision to my staff, do I worry about what the staff will think and say about me (more than what they will think and say about the decision)?

✔ When I report an unpopular decision, do I usually say, "I didn't have anything to do with this," "It's not my fault," or another "Don't get mad at me" statement?

✔ Do I back down from enforcing policies because I do not want to deal with the resentment of the staff?

✔ When I make the work schedule, am I guided first by my interest in serving the needs of my staff (rather than my commitment to serving our patients/clients)?

✔ Do I subtly try to align my staff with me against my supervisor?

✔ Do I speak negatively about my supervisor to my staff?

✔ Do I find myself trying to do my staff's work to gain their acceptance/approval?

✔ Are my efforts to help my staff with their work impeding my ability to meet the requirements of *my* job?

✔ Do I avoid terminating an employee when it is necessary?

✔ Do I show favoritism to any member of my staff?

✔ Do I give good performance evaluations to all my staff regardless of performance?

✔ Is it clear to my staff how they can earn "perks," such as extra education days, bonuses, or other privileges?

✔ Do I strike a balance between lending hands-on assistance to my staff and managing my department so that my staff does not routinely need this assistance?

✔ Do I provide ample opportunity for my staff to express their concerns and needs?

✔ Whenever possible, do I request input from my staff in making decisions that affect our department?

✔ Do I ask for input from my staff on things they would like to see change in our department?

✔ Do I clearly explain how much change I can and cannot effect?

✔ Whenever possible, do I request input from my staff in determining how to execute management decisions?

✔ Do I set clear verbal and written expectations and goals for my staff?

✔ When an employee does not meet expectations, do I provide clear verbal and written guidelines and expectations for improvement?

✔ Do I understand and follow human resource guidelines in taking disciplinary action with members of my staff?

✔ If I take disciplinary action against an employee, is it the same action I would take against *any* employee with the same record?

The first 11 questions address fundamentals of your responsibility as a nurse manager and your ability to execute these basics effectively. If you responded "yes" to any of these questions, you may be resisting the psychologic jump from staff nurse to nurse manager. Or you may need additional guidance or training in effective management. Take a serious look at your thinking and your management practices. You probably need to adjust both. If you answered "no" to these questions, you have a good start in defining your role as a nurse manager.

The rest of the questions address your ability to (1) facilitate open communication with your staff and (2) create a fair, supportive work environment. A "yes" response to these questions indicates a commitment to these goals. If you answered "no" to any of these questions, consider the consequences of your management practice in question. For example, if you fail to set clear guidelines for performance improvement, it will be difficult for an employee to meet your expectations. You will create a stressful work environment—one in which an employee may never really understand what you expect. Or, if you fail to follow human resource guidelines for disciplinary action, you will create an unpredictable and stressful work environment. In addition, your disciplinary actions may be overturned in grievance procedures, greatly weakening your credibility. As you examine the consequences of your management practices, you will probably realize that the energy you invest to create a predictable, positive workplace will pay great dividends.

How the Manager Views the Staff

The way the manager views the staff is generally given less attention than the way the staff views the manager. Just as a certain authority is vested in the manager, the manager enters this role with beliefs about employees. These beliefs vary, depending on the manager.

For example, some managers may view their employees as children to be cajoled, scolded, rescued, and praised. Some managers may view their employees as threats to their jobs, people who potentially could unseat them. Other managers may view their employees as a group of potential friends and supporters who will meet their emotional needs for love and acceptance.

Ideally, a manager will view employees as valuable members of the team—a group of people who can cooperate in creating a successful work environment. Although the manager must provide guidance, leadership, and support, her self-respect and respect for the employees will not falter.

How a manager views her staff generally depends more on the psychologic make-up of the manager and less on the actual history or potential of the staff. Because of this, it is important to assess your beliefs before you get too far into your job. The more you understand about how you view your staff, the easier it will be for you to avoid intensifying stress and creating problems with your staff. Also, this understanding will help you identify problems for what they really are, not for what you may believe them to be.

For example, if you are the type of manager who tends to view your staff as children, you may unknowingly create stress and resentment among the ranks. Few adults want to be treated like a child.

If you feel threatened by your staff, not only will this be evident to the staff, your management judgment will be impaired. It's difficult to make fair decisions and carry out your responsibilities if you're preoccupied with protecting your own interests.

If you view your staff as potential friends, you may create an adolescent environment with an "in crowd" and an "out crowd." This is not effective in the adult world of providing services to patients, carrying out responsibilities, and building careers.

Although these examples of manager beliefs may be ineffective and sometimes even destructive, most managers enter their roles with a little of each of these, as well as other points of view. What is important is that you understand how you actually *do* see your staff—before you determine how you think you *should* see your staff.

As you determine how you actually see your employees, you are in a better position to change your point of view, if necessary, and to develop effective management practices.

Ideally, you come to your manager role with a healthy respect for your staff and yourself—a respect that all human beings deserve, whether they are one of the best nurses in town or one of those who needs help developing. On this premise you can build a realistic and effective view of your staff—one in which stress is manageable and all are able to thrive.

Inventory of Your Beliefs About Your Staff

Below are questions to help you clarify your management practices regarding your beliefs about or preconceived notions of your staff. They are designed as triggers to help you think and develop or change your beliefs.

Following the inventory are guidelines for you to evaluate your responses to the first eight questions. The rest of the questions will help you reflect on how comfortable and confident you are in your role and in "what makes you tick" as a nurse manager.

BELIEFS ABOUT YOUR STAFF—QUESTIONS TO ASK YOURSELF

✔ Do I invite feedback from my staff?

✔ Do I invite constructive criticism of management policies or practices, including my own?

✔ Do I communicate my staff's concerns to my supervisor?

✔ Do I discuss star performers with my supervisor? Do I discuss problem employees with my supervisor?

✔ Do I communicate openly with my staff about the overall operations and goals of the institution or business? Whenever possible, do I inform them of any information handed down to me?

✔ Am I easily irritated when my staff expresses dissatisfaction with a policy or management practice? Why?

✔ Do I discuss staff members' personal or work-related problems with other staff members? Why?

✔ Are there staff members to whom I give preferential treatment? Why?

✔ Do I think someone on my staff wants my job? Why do I think this? Would this person or someone else on my staff be able to do my job? What have I done to explore her professional growth objectives? What have I done to encourage capable staff members to consider a management job in this institution or elsewhere?

✔ What do I think of my previous managers? Was anyone exceptionally good? Exceptionally poor? Why?

✔ How did my previous managers view their staffs? Do I share any of these views? How did their opinions of their staffs affect the staffs? Were the managers' opinions of their staffs justified? Why do I think this? Did their opinions of their staffs become self-fulfilling prophesies? Why do I think this?

✔ What are the positive lessons I have learned from my previous managers? How can I incorporate these lessons into my management style?

✔ What aspects of my previous managers' styles do I want to avoid? Why? How can I avoid repeating management practices that could be mistakes?

✔ How do I think my present supervisor views me? Is this justified? Why? Is this effective and productive? Why?

✔ Do I want to pass on this view of subordinates to my staff? Why? How can I do or not do this?

"Yes" responses to the first five questions generally indicate a positive, respectful attitude toward your staff.

If you respond "yes" to any of the next three questions, you may be experiencing problems with your management role (i.e., recognizing the boundaries between you and your staff, as well as recognizing your responsibility to be objective and fair). For example, if you find you are generally irritated when your staff is dissatisfied, you may be personalizing their reactions. Your irritation may stem from your own difficulties in recognizing boundaries.

COPING MECHANISMS

Although many sources of stress are in the nursing workplace, individual nurses cope differently with these stresses.

In their study of critical care nurses, Robinson and Lewis[5] reviewed various coping mechanisms, including adaptive and maladaptive mechanisms. Adaptive coping mechanisms are positive responses to stress and require no intervention. Maladaptive coping mechanisms indicate a negative response to stress and call for stress management intervention.

COPING MECHANISMS IDENTIFIED BY ROBINSON AND LEWIS[5]

✔ Take vacation

✔ Watch television or read

✔ Problem solving

✔ Hobbies

✔ Discuss problems with family

✔ Caffeine (coffee, tea, or soft drinks)

✔ Exercise

✔ Consider changing jobs

✔ Work harder and enjoy less

✔ Overeating

✔ Progressive relaxation techniques

✔ Deny problems

✔ Alcohol

✔ Absenteeism

✔ Imagery

✔ Meditation

✔ Smoking

✔ Self-hypnosis

✔ Drugs to relax

✔ Discuss problems with coworkers

As you can see, this list includes adaptive and maladaptive coping mechanisms. Although the study characterized various mechanisms as either adaptive or maladaptive, some of these coping mechanisms could fall into either category. For example, discussing problems with one's family may prove to be adaptive for one individual but maladaptive for another.

The way a nurse copes with stress in the workplace is highly individualized. Coping mechanisms that work for one may not work for another. In addition, a coping mechanism that works for a nurse under low-level stress may not work for that same nurse under higher levels of stress.

For the purposes of this discussion, those coping mechanisms which cause additional, albeit different, physical or emotional stress in a nurse are maladaptive coping mechanisms. Generally, behaviors such as overeating, overworking, drinking alcohol, smoking, and so forth eventually cause additional stress in the nurse.

Stress Evaluation Exercise: Coping Mechanisms

Earlier in this chapter, you were asked to list as many sources of stress in your work environment as you could identify. As a follow-up to this exercise, now list all coping mechanisms you can imagine. Do not exclude those coping mechanisms you consider to be maladaptive. After generating your coping mechanisms list, consider those coping mechanisms which may be helpful and those which may not be helpful. Identify reasons some coping mechanisms may be adaptive and some maladaptive. You may further define coping mechanisms in terms of their usefulness for various levels of stress (e.g., taking a vacation may be appropriate as temporary relief from long-term stress, and reading or watching television may be effective as relief from short-term stress brought on by a rough day).

If you are doing this exercise with some of your peers, take ample time for discussion. Resist the temptation to push your personal agenda. Rather, learn from each other and broaden your understanding of how people cope with stress.

UNMANAGED STRESS IN THE NURSING WORKPLACE

Recognizing the signs of unmanaged stress in the workplace is critical to the nurse manager's ability to respond constructively to her own and the staff's needs.

Understanding the sources of stress in the nursing workplace and the accompanying coping mechanisms is a prerequisite to understanding what you and your staff are experiencing. When a stressful situation continues for an extended period, or when coping mechanisms are maladaptive or are failing, stress may become unmanageable.

Unfortunately, early signs—and even later signs—of unmanaged stress often go unnoticed. In fact, some managers first recognize that stress is spiraling out of control when the staff resigns in legion numbers. Staff members themselves may not even recognize the early signs.

For various reasons, nurse managers often fail to recognize early stress signals. Most managers have risen through the nursing ranks. They have often been conditioned by their supervisors to ignore stress until it reaches mountainous proportions. Thus, "It's always been like this," becomes a way to minimize the seriousness of stressful situations. Some nurse managers bring to their jobs a history of ignoring their own signs and symptoms of unmanaged stress, as well as inexperience in recognizing others' signs of unmanaged stress. In addition, the new nurse manager has not had the experience of viewing stress from the vantage point of a manager and claiming responsibility for helping the staff to manage it.

Breakwell,[6] in analyzing the stresses experienced by those in the health care profession, discusses the effects of stress as being both psychologic and behavioral. The psychologic effects are seen in changes in one's thinking, as well as in one's emotions.

EFFECTS OF UNMANAGED STRESS

Some changes in thinking described by Breakwell.[6]

✔ Deteriorating memory

✔ Declining concentration and attention span

✔ Dissipating powers of organization and long-term planning

Some emotional changes.

✔ Depression

✔ Hostility

✔ Defensiveness

✔ Feelings of powerlessness and worthlessness

✔ Cynicism

✔ Mood swings

✔ Hypochondria

✔ Personality changes (e.g., a shy person becomes gregarious or vice-versa)

Some behavioral effects of stress.

✔ Decreased energy level

✔ Disrupted sleep

✔ Increased drinking and/or smoking

✔ Absenteeism from work

✔ Diminished sex drive

✔ Lack of enthusiasm

✔ Lack of interest in activities and hobbies that once were satisfying

Wilson[7] warns that the changes brought on by chronic, unrelieved stress may be subtle.

✔ Feeling overwhelmed

✔ Fatigue, angry outbursts, depression

✔ Forgetfulness and disorganization

✔ Guilt and self-sacrifice

✔ Feeling disillusioned

✔ Passivity

✔ Distancing yourself from your patients

✔ Letting yourself go

✔ Substance abuse

✔ Physical illness

Stress Evaluation Exercise: Signs of Unmanaged Stress

Nurse managers would do well to monitor themselves and their staffs for the changes brought on by unmanaged stress. Because many of these changes are subjective symptoms, astute nurse managers must learn to observe staff members for the objective signs that usually accompany these subjective symptoms. See the accompanying box for a stress inventory checklist.

FAILING TO MANAGE STRESS: A COMMON PITFALL

Once a nurse manager learns to identify signs of stress in the workplace, the next step is problem solving and responding to this stress. Failing to respond constructively to stress in the workplace is a common pitfall for nurse managers.

Often managers minimize the toll stress can take on themselves and their staffs, ignoring even late warning signs of stress's wear and tear. There are many reasons for this failing. For example, a nurse manager may ignore the effects of stress because of a fear of impotence (e.g., "There's nothing I can do about it, so I'll ignore it."). Unfortunately, this attitude of impotence—no matter how toughly exhibited—is communicated to the staff. When one experiences impo-

STAFF STRESS INVENTORY CHECKLIST

Managers can take stock of what they are seeing in their staffs' behavior by asking themselves questions that address Wilson's[7] list of symptoms. You may ask yourself the questions in reference to an individual on the staff or in regard to the staff as a whole. For the purposes of this discussion, assume that you are considering one individual.

FEELING OVERWHELMED

Is she slow to start at the beginning of the workday?_____
Does she "jump right in," before having had the chance to organize the
  workday? _____
Does she dart from task to task without a clear sense of purpose or control?_____
Does she seem to respond mostly to the "squeaky wheel" (or patient), rather than
  acting on priorities?_____
Does she express a fatalistic attitude about the workload, (e.g., "Oh well, it's not
  going to get done anyway.")?_____
Does she consistently have to work overtime to complete assignments?_____
Has she failed to complete assignments?_____

FATIGUE, ANGRY OUTBURSTS, AND DEPRESSION

Does he lose his temper at the slightest provocation?_____
Does he respond rudely or abruptly to patients?_____
Is he rough with patients?_____
Has he become quiet or unusually reserved?_____
Has he lost his sense of humor? _____
Does he get tearful with little provocation? _____
Does he remark that the job is "getting to him."?_____
Has he been absent from work more often than is considered average
  absenteeism?_____
Does he say he is depressed?_____
Has he shown personality changes?_____
Has he become disinterested or apathetic about work?_____
Has he become disinterested or apathetic about other aspects of his life? _____

FORGETFULNESS AND DISORGANIZATION

Is she making more than the normal amount of mistakes?_____
Are you seeing an increase in her incident reports? _____
Does she forget aspects of patient care? _____
Does she forget to report patient problems appropriately?_____
Is she failing to recognize patient problems or to make logical deductions about pa-
  tient problems? _____
Are her usual thinking abilities impaired? _____
Does she seem distracted?_____
When you address her, does she sometimes seem not to hear you? _____

Continued

STAFF STRESS INVENTORY CHECKLIST—cont'd

GUILT AND SELF-SACRIFICE

Is he coming to work when he is ill?_____
Is he consistently skipping lunch or work breaks to catch up on work? _____
Is he consistently working overtime? _____
Does he consistently volunteer for distasteful tasks, overtime assignments, and holiday shifts?_____

FEELING DISILLUSIONED

Does she express resentment about the nursing profession?_____
Does she express envy of people in other professions or regret that she became a nurse? _____
Does she remark that the actual practice of nursing is much different from what she learned in school? _____
Does she express regret that she can never deliver the type of care she would like to deliver?_____
Does she express feelings of hopelessness about nursing (e.g., "It will never change.")?_____

PASSIVITY

Does he take abuse from coworkers or physicians?_____
Does he remark that "it's not worth" disagreeing with difficult individuals?_____
Does he seem indifferent about problem-solving?_____
Is he among the first people you consider when you must assign a distasteful task (because you know there will be no resistance)?_____
Is he described as a wimp by coworkers?_____

DISTANCING ONESELF FROM PATIENTS

Does she refer to patients as disease entities, rather than as people (e.g., "the hepatitis in 22.")? _____
Does she respond irritably to patients who "interrupt" tasks with questions or requests? _____
Does she limit conversation with patients by speaking only when absolutely necessary?_____
Does she ask patients to make their requests all at once so she can limit interactions with them?_____
Does she focus almost exclusively on the physical aspects of caring for patients, rather than also considering the psychologic aspects? _____
Does she make remarks about family members who "interfere" with patient care by asking questions or making requests?_____
Is she "cold" or "cool" to patients? _____

LETTING ONESELF GO

Has he gained or lost weight recently?_____
Is his appearance sloppy or haphazard?_____

STAFF STRESS INVENTORY CHECKLIST—cont'd

SUBSTANCE ABUSE

Is she drinking more coffee or smoking more cigarettes?_____
Has she said she is taking something to sleep?_____
Has she been late to work?_____
Has she been absent from work more often than is considered average absenteeism? _____
Has she joked or commented about excessive "partying"?_____
Is she showing any of the physical or psychologic signs of chemical dependency?_____ (Refer to later section, "When You Identify A Serious Staff Problem.")

PHYSICAL ILLNESS

Has he had excessive absenteeism because of illness?_____
Does he seem to have an inordinate number of colds, headaches, or gastrointestinal problems?_____

Adapted from Wilson LK: High-gear nursing: how it can run you down and what you can do about it, *Nursing '89,* 19(12):81, 1989.

tence in the face of stress, the stress is magnified, creating an even more strained environment. On the contrary, the sense that one can effect change, regardless of degree, provides a feeling of hope and empowerment.

A second reason nurse managers may fail to respond constructively to stress is a false sense of their own invulnerability. This sense of invulnerability—"That doesn't bother me," "I've been in nursing 10 years (or 3 or 5 years), I'm used to that,"—often is no more than a way of building up to the burnout so many nurses experience. A nurse who appears immune to the emotional roller coaster of nursing may in fact be closer to burnout than suspected.

For example, distancing oneself from and depersonalizing patients (e.g., "the colon cancer in 13-A" or "the three 'total-cares' I had today") help a nurse avoid feelings of frustration, fear, or grief but are poor substitutes for accepting and sharing these feelings with others.

In the long run, trying to be invulnerable leaves one vulnerable to frustration, depression, and burnout. And a nurse manager who, by example, fosters such invulnerability in her staff also fosters burnout in her staff.

A third reason nurse managers may fail to respond constructively to stress is a misguided belief that managers are expected to "roll with"—rather than respond to—stressful situations. Often managers are concerned that acknowledgement of the stress level in their area may indicate a deficiency in their management skills. This concern is heightened when a manager's own supervisor appears unaware or invulnerable to stress.

You may be able to identify other reasons nurses and nurse managers fail to respond constructively to stress. Regardless of the explanation, the result is the same: failure to respond constructively to stress leads to increased stress. When you are able to recognize unmanaged stress, you are better able to respond to stress in the workplace with effective coping mechanisms. You will also be better equipped to respond to the needs of your staff and help them in enhancing their adaptive coping mechanisms.

WHEN YOU IDENTIFY A SERIOUS STAFF PROBLEM

Occasionally you will identify an employee who has a serious problem. This problem may be caused by job stress, personal difficulties, or a combination of factors.

If you are concerned that an employee's performance may be impaired because of chemical dependence, or that she may be experiencing serious emotional problems or depression, you need to request guidance. You can speak with your employee assistance program (EAP) counselor, the staff social worker or psychologist, the psychiatric nurse specialist, or a professional outside your organization.

It generally is best to use your organization's resources first. People within your organization may know the employee, or your organization may have resources or policies to respond to these types of problems.

If you do seek assistance from an outside professional to guide you in your dealings with an employee, resources are usually available. Most cities have emergency or crisis hotlines for referrals to appropriate organizations, many of which will discuss your concerns about your employee free of charge. Hospital emergency rooms frequently keep hotline and other organization listings.

Discuss your concerns with your supervisor and determine a course of action. If your supervisor is not responsive, these cases—because of their serious nature and possible consequences—obligate you to take your concerns up your organization's chain of command or to HR, the EAP counselor, or other professional until you get assistance.

The Chemically Dependent Employee

It is important for nurse managers to be aware of the problems of alcohol and other chemical dependencies in the health professions. Bissell,[8] a nationally recognized expert on addicted health care professionals, and Jones[8] conducted research indicating the severity of chemical dependency in the nursing profession. Their research suggests that approximately 5% of the 1.5 million registered nurses in the United States are dependent on alcohol and/or drugs.

Selbach[9] cites job strain—including factors such as the nursing shortage, work overload, and dealing with illness and death—as a source of the frustration and stress contributing to a nurse becoming chemically dependent. She cites rotating shifts, night duty, chronic stress, tension, fatigue, and anxiety as factors that can lead to insomnia and the initial use of chemicals to unwind, relax, and sleep. In addition, most nurses are women, and many actually have two full-time jobs, nurse and mother, and try to be "superwoman" at both.

A word of caution: the chemically dependent nurse, like many others dependent on drugs or alcohol, often does not embody the stereotype of the debilitated addict. In fact, some chemically dependent nurses are excellent workers who show no sign of their dependency until late in the disease. The chemically dependent nurse may be a high achiever, an individual who has done well in school and in past jobs and may have been the model employee/spouse/friend/parent before the dependency. She often is a compulsive individual, which is a trait that can lend itself to good patient care but which can also cause the nurse to create unrealistic expectations of herself at work and in other areas of life. These expectations can produce the stress overload the nurse believes is alleviated by using drugs and/or alcohol. See the box on pg. 237 for signs of the chemically dependent nurse.

Many health care facilities have policies concerning the chemically dependent employee, including policies to assist the employee in seeking treatment. Although terminating a chemically dependent employee may appear to be a quick fix, the terminated employee probably will not seek treatment. In fact, she will probably move onto another job—the "geographic cure"—taking the chemical dependency into another workplace.

As a nurse manager facing the possibility of a chemically dependent employee, your responsibilities are two-fold: (1) to see that your patients are receiving proper care from responsible employees and (2) to address the needs of the chemically dependent employee, including the right to privacy and the opportunity to seek help.

SIGNS OF THE CHEMICALLY DEPENDENT NURSE

Numbers 1 through 7 are signs identified by Patton, an occupational health nurse and EAP coordinator. Other common signs follow.
1. Too many medication errors.
2. Frequent absences from the nursing unit.
3. Too many controlled substances wasted and/or spilled.
4. Consistently incorrect narcotics count.
5. Signs out more controlled substances than do others.
6. Rapid, extreme, and inappropriate mood changes.
7. Patient complaints of the ineffectiveness of pain medication when administered by individual. (This could be a sign that the nurse is substituting saline or sterile water, emptying capsules, or substituting nonnarcotic tablets.)
8. Excessive absenteeism.
9. Tardiness.
10. Getting by at work, but not performing beyond the bare minimum needed.
11. Failure to complete assignments.
12. Leaving responsibilities to other staff.
13. Sloppy, illogical, nonexistent, or meaningless charting (often by rote and could apply to any patient).
14. Excessive incident reports and/or failure to file incident reports.
15. Excessive mistakes.
16. Abnormal physiologic reactions resulting from drug or alcohol use, such as headaches, diarrhea, lack of sleep, and withdrawal symptoms.
17. Inappropriate behavior or quick flashes of temper.
18. Personality changes.
19. Obvious physical signs of drug use, such as slurring speech, rapid speech, smell of alcohol, confusion, or weight loss.
20. Accusations that people are "out to get" or are against her.
21. Blaming others and refusal to take responsibility for actions.

Reprinted with permission from Patton J: Addicted nurses, *J Pract Nurs* 37(4):40, 1987.

If you believe you have a chemically dependent employee on your staff, discuss the matter with your supervisor to determine a course of action (i.e., what policies your organization has in place, what professional person will guide you). If your supervisor is not responsive, continue to seek guidance.

The Employee with Emotional Difficulties

If you are concerned that an employee is severely depressed, disturbed, or suicidal, seek guidance immediately to determine how to handle the situation. If you have fears or concerns that an employee is "not right," these feelings are probably well founded. In these cases, you must provide for the safety of your patients and determine, with the help of your supervisor and a trained professional, how to support your employee. Again, if your supervisor is not responsive to your concern, seek guidance from others.

Other Serious Problems

Aside from chemical dependency and emotional difficulties, other serious problems that warrant attention may manifest themselves in your department as a whole or in a member or members of your staff. For instance, sometimes a staff copes with stress by blaming you, another individual on the staff, or a small group of individuals for the stress. This scapegoating can become a way of life in the department and can devastate the person or persons being scapegoated. In addition, it never alleviates the stress in the department because it does not solve the problem.

Other problems that may arise in your department could affect almost everyone on your staff. The situation may be the result of long-term problems within your organization or department, such as excessive turnover, or it may be a problem that is clearly time-limited—whether it be 1 month or 1 year in duration. Examples of these situations include major management changes (e.g., a new CEO who effects many changes), a large construction or renovation project that disrupts daily activities, a flu epidemic that depletes the staff, or the introduction of computerized scheduling, which requires a period of adjustment while the "bugs" are worked out.

In some instances, you may recognize that many of your staff are experiencing a great deal of stress, but you can not identify the source. If you think your staff as a group is feeling the strain of unmanaged stress, regardless of the source, it may be helpful to invite a professional to facilitate an ongoing staff support group. It is not recommended that a nurse manager try to lead these group meetings. The support group should allow for the sharing of feelings and personal interpretations, which only a trained professional should direct. In addition, if there are communication gaps between you and any of your staff members, a professional can help in closing these gaps. Discuss your options with your supervisor.

UNMANAGEABLE ENVIRONMENTS

Although most problems can be solved with time and the proper guidance and intervention, you may find yourself in a work environment in which the problems are so many or so deeply rooted that you are unable to be an effective manager. In this instance, it is generally best for you to leave the position.

There are many understandable reasons why you may leave a job. Some examples include a poor job match for you, a disagreement with the values or policies of a supervisor or organization, a realization that you prefer not to be a manager, or a realization that you are not ready to be a manager. Another understandable reason for leaving a job is the recognition that you are attempting to manage an unmanageable environment.

Generally, an unmanageable environment is characterized by two components: (1) a serious problem exists in the department or organization, and (2) you have little or ineffective management support in solving it. If your immediate supervisor shows little support or if her support is ineffective, you may be able to find help from someone else within your organization. Some problems, because of their serious nature, require you to seek this help when your immediate supervisor is not responsive. Some of these situations were discussed earlier in this chapter, under "When You Identify a Serious Staff Problem."

You may identify other serious problems that call for immediate attention. For instance, staffing that is so lean that patient care is threatened would require you to seek help beyond a nonresponsive supervisor.

A word of caution: when you secure problem-solving assistance or intervention from someone in your organization other than your supervisor, the immediate problem may be resolved, but you have not changed your environment. Although your first responsibility must be to solve the immediate problem, you must then evaluate your options and the viability of continuing as a manager with an ineffective supervisor.

Ineffective Management Support

A supervisor may demonstrate ineffective management support or a lack of management support to the nurse manager in many ways. For example, the nurse manager may be restricted from taking corrective action against employees who defy the policies of the organization or department. The manager may be prevented from taking disciplinary action against an employee who is rough with a patient. The supervisor may listen sympathetically to the nurse manager's concerns about the department, but offer no advice or direction. The nurse manager may be consistently scapegoated by the staff, and the supervisor may offer no guidance for dealing with this situation.

These are a few examples of how a supervisor may fail to support a nurse manager. In each case, the manager's inability to take action, to correct a problem, or to establish leadership authority will affect the morale of the staff, the quality of patient care, and the manager's ability to manage the department.

Sometimes a new nurse manager enters a job without knowledge of the department's history and resulting problems. Perhaps the staff believes the previous manager was unfairly dismissed from the position. Or they may have experienced a long period without leadership and resent the arrival of the new manager. These factors alone do not necessarily create an unmanageable environment. However, if the new nurse manager receives little support and guidance from her supervisor, effective management could be difficult.

Combined with ineffective support or a lack of support from management above you, the following is a list of conditions that could signal an unmanageable environment. You may be able to add items to this list. Included in the list are some additional destructive behaviors your supervisor could exhibit—behaviors that go beyond not showing support and are more actively destructive.

SIGNS OF AN UNMANAGEABLE ENVIRONMENT

✔ An individual or group (or clique) of nurses holding the unspoken power in the division.

✔ Understaffing, with no plan or hope for improvement.

✔ Poor patient care.

✔ Staff scapegoating of you or a member of your staff.

✔ A chemically dependent employee.

✔ An employee stealing drugs, narcotics, or supplies.

✔ Widespread absenteeism.

✔ An employee coming in late to work, leaving early, or disappearing during the work day.

✔ An employee who physically or emotionally abuses patients.

✔ An employee who defies the policies of the organization.

✔ An employee who shows you no respect (e.g., walking away from you when you talk, shouting at you, ignoring you).

✔ A staff that is divided along lines of race, gender, professional status, levels of competence, tenure, or other factors.

✔ A supervisor who makes management decisions based on any of the factors cited in the preceding point.

✔ A supervisor who maintains friendships with one or more staff members who do not support you or who undermine your authority.

✔ A supervisor who misrepresents you to upper management (e.g., lying about you, taking credit for your work).

✔ A supervisor who listens to the complaints of the staff (about you, your management, or other matters related to your department) without encouraging the staff to talk to you and/or without informing you of the conversations.

✔ An apathetic staff.

✔ An employee who defies your instructions, policies, and so forth.

✔ An employee who seems seriously depressed, disturbed, or suicidal.

✔ Other conditions you have identified.

If you determine that you are in an unmanageable environment, it is important that you give yourself permission to resign your position. Sometimes nurse managers are reluctant to give up on a job, believing if they only try harder, conditions will improve. In an unmanageable environment, unfortunately, this often is not the case. By definition, this type of environment cannot be improved without radical changes in the leadership above.

If you resign a position because you believe the work environment to be unmanageable, you may want to request an exit interview with an objective nurse recruiter, personnel director, or other individual in an influential position who may be receptive to listening. Each organization is different, and you will have to determine your best course. Because patient care may be at stake, it is important to share your perceptions of the environment in the hope that the situation will be addressed. As you relate your perceptions, take care to provide only the facts, not your subjective feelings or intuitions about the situation. For example, relate problematic events in your department and how you attempted to get help to solve them.

Sometimes it is best to schedule an exit interview for a time after you have recovered from the immediate stress of your resignation. If you choose to pursue an exit interview, it will be important for you to conduct the interview calmly, presenting your information in a rational manner.

TAKING ACTION TO SUPPORT YOUR STAFF

Fortunately, most nurse managers do not find themselves in unmanageable environments. And in most cases, there are many steps a nurse manager can take to alleviate routine stress in her department. Everyone agrees that a nurse manager's support is critical to the staff's successful management of stress. Albrecht and Halsey[10] suggest that we consider "social support as verbal and nonverbal communication between recipients and providers, which reduces uncertainty about the situation, the self, and others . . . to enhance personal control."

Albrecht and Halsey Study on Support to Staff Nurses

Albrecht and Halsey[10] discuss the types of messages that are most helpful to a distressed nurse.

*HELPFUL MESSAGES FOR THE DISTRESSED NURSE**

✔ Reduce uncertainty by offering a new perspective on the problem (e.g., "Why don't you think about this?).

✔ Help increase feelings of control over the problem by allowing education days or teaching new skills.

*Modified from Albrecht TL, Halsey J: Supporting the staff nurse under stress, Nurs Manage 22(7):60, 1991.

> ✔ Help enhance a sense of control over the problem by providing tangible assistance (in a friendly, noncondescending manner).
>
> ✔ Offer acceptance and reassurance.

Albrecht's and Halsey's study[10] of staff nurses' stress and how their managers support them was very revealing. The nurses' perceptions of a manager's supportive behaviors were measured separately in four hypothetical stress situations. The combined results show that the manager's listening, offering reassurance, or giving advice were supportive behaviors that were valued by many of the nurses. Although the manager's taking action to solve the problem also was viewed as supportive, the results showed that this behavior was not valued by as many nurses as were the manager's communication and advising behaviors.

However, one stress situation in which many of the nurses viewed the manager's action as supportive was when the staff nurses were working in an understaffed situation. Here, the manager's helping with the work was particularly valued. This makes sense because understaffing threatens the nurses' ability to provide good patient care, the driving desire of most nurses. However, even in this situation, many nurses also valued the manager's listening skills.

As a nurse manager, you must weigh each stressful situation and determine the steps you can take to support your staff. In some instances, active, as well as communicative support, is imperative, lest you become known for "all talk and no action." In the case of understaffing, it may be important to help in the immediate situation, then take action to see that understaffing does not become a chronic problem.

The lesson to be learned from Albrecht's and Halsey's study[10] is not to underestimate the value of each of a manager's methods of offering support to the staff: listening, offering reassurance, giving advice, taking action, validating your staff's feelings, and helping your staff understand the perspective of other employees and of physicians.

In some cases, good communication skills or concrete suggestions will greatly alleviate staff nurses' stress. In others, you will need to combine this support with action.

To address some forms of stress, you may need to make changes in how your department operates. Be mindful of ways you can alter your work environment to alleviate stress. Include your staff in discussions of ways to modify operations for a smoother, less stressful work day. Enlist the guidance and support of your supervisor. Work with your supervisor to determine what changes you can and cannot effect and why. For example, if you have been unable to fill some vacant positions, what alternatives do you have to tide the staff over until the positions are filled? Is there a way to get more secretarial support? Can you employ temporary nurses? Can you draw more help from the float pool? Are there some non–patient care activities that can be suspended until your positions are filled?

Drawing on the Work and Experience of Other Nurse Managers

Many nurse managers fall into the trap of thinking they are alone in dealing with staff stress. In addition to your supervisor and a myriad of other resource people within and outside your organization, consider the experience of your peers. Ask them how they support their staffs and consider if these techniques would work for your staff. Be sensitive to the differences in departments, personnel, and your personality versus the personalities of your peers. What works for them may not work for you. Also, you may find that you simply do not agree with the approaches of some of your peers. Nonetheless, your peer group may offer new ways of looking at conditions and new ideas for supporting your staff.

Another resource to consider is the nursing literature. Much has been written about stress in nursing and the allied health care professions. A trip to a nursing or medical library can result in a lot of new information. If you have specific concerns, such as the impaired nurse or the stress of dealing with death and dying, you can easily find articles on these topics. If there is no nursing or medical library in your facility or where you live, contact your local library to see if they carry any appropriate journals. Also, if your organization has an education or training department, consult with the director.

Subscribing to one or more of the nursing professional journals is a good idea, both for the clinical and management information. You may want to share subscriptions with some of your peers to cut costs and increase your access to various publications.

Communicating with Upper Management

An important way to support your staff is to communicate their concerns to your supervisor. By working with your supervisor, you may be able to generate additional ways to demonstrate support to your staff.

If your department is experiencing a particularly stressful situation, be certain to let them know that you and your supervisor are concerned. Tell the staff what you and your supervisor are able to do to support them. Often, your staff's knowing that you recognize their stress is the first step in alleviating it. Also, their knowing that you consider their feelings important enough to discuss with your supervisor lets them know that you care.

Humor

Humor can break the tension in even the most stressful situation. If you are attuned to the sensitivities of your staff and have a good sense of timing, you can use humor very effectively to make a tough day a little less stressful.

As wonderful as humor can be, there are some basic guidelines concerning its use. For example, never make a joke at the expense of another person—present or absent—or at the expense of a group of people based on their gender, race, sexual orientation, and so on, regardless of whether a member of the group is on your staff. Hostile, bigoted, or demeaning humor may lead to feelings of insecurity among your staff (e.g., "When will she come after me or someone like me?").

In addition, it is important not to use humor at an inappropriate time, such as in a serious patient-care situation that requires concentration. Laughter at this time could have serious consequences for the patient. Also, do not use any form of humor that would show disrespect for a patient or his family.

Particularly effective is light-hearted humor poking fun at yourself (however, not at your gender, race, sexual orientation, and so forth). If you are comfortable with self-deprecating humor, you can give your staff the chance to relax a little, as well as to see you in a more personal light, thus strengthening the bonds between you. According to Lee,[11] "Team spirit and improved staff morale are benefits reaped by the nurse manager who knows how to take her job seriously while taking herself lightly."

Lee[11] notes that it is difficult for most people to tell a scripted joke and get the desired effect, particularly to a group or to people with whom relationships are not well developed. For spontaneous situations, Lee suggests that a comical remark about a personal event or predicament generally works best.

TIPS FOR LENDING SUPPORT TO YOUR STAFF

✔ Encourage camaraderie among your staff. Provide the opportunity for them to know each other as people, not just as nurses. Whenever possible, schedule breaks and meals for at least two nurses at a time.

✔ Sponsor a staff party away from the workplace a few times a year. A pot-luck dinner is an inexpensive way to get together and will encourage staff participation.

✔ Take time to know your staff. Ask about their families, friends, and school experiences. Take some of your breaks and meals with them.

✔ Let your staff know you. Do not discourage casual conversation. Let them know it is okay to ask you about yourself by volunteering information about your life and interests away from the job. However, do not overdo it by talking about yourself in a one-sided conversation.

✔ Allow time at regular staff meetings for your employees to ask questions and voice concerns. You can invite this communication broadly (e.g., "Is there anything anyone would like to discuss?") and specifically (e.g., "Does anyone have any questions or concerns about our new admissions policy?"). A combination of both techniques is most effective.

✔ Recognize unmanaged stress (e.g., "It seems this is a difficult time," "Are you okay?" "It would make sense that you would be stressed out today.").

✔ Listen. Listen. And listen again.

✔ If you are concerned that someone may be experiencing stress, talk to the person and offer reassurance and support with constructive problem-solving. In cases of severe stress, look to your supervisor and a trained professional for guidance.

✔ Provide time in the workday for your staff to think and reflect on the best way to organize and deliver their patient care.

✔ Provide regular staff in-services and updating of skills.

✔ Allow for education days for your staff to encourage them to develop professionally.

✔ Use your supervisor for assistance in supporting your staff.

✔ Help your staff learn to manage their time.

✔ Arrange staff coverage so that your employees are able to take vacation breaks on a regular basis.

✔ Offer words of support, recognizing your staff's good work and giving positive feedback frequently and freely.

SUPPORTING YOURSELF

As was discussed at the beginning of this chapter, it is critical that you support yourself as you simultaneously support your staff from the effects of stress. Listed later are various ways to help you manage long-term and short-term job stress. However, there are individuals for whom these and other methods may not work. The following discussion addresses these individuals.

If you believe your environment is basically manageable, but you are having difficulty coping with the stress of your job, give yourself permission to get professional help, either from your EAP counselor, another in-house professional, or a professional counselor or therapist outside your organization. Remember, you are new to your job and to the stresses of being a manager. Even when you are an experienced nurse manager, there may come a time when you feel your coping mechanisms are failing you. Do not consider yourself inadequate if you are having problems dealing with the stress of your job. Discussing your situation with an impartial professional can help you to problem-solve, strengthen your coping mechanisms, or develop new ones.

If There Is No Hope in Sight

You may reach a point where you cannot handle the stresses of your job, despite the fact that the environment may be manageable (when viewed objectively), despite your best efforts to problem-solve and seek help, and despite your belief that you should be able to handle the stress. Or you simply may know it is best for you to leave your position because you are not able or do not want to invest the energy necessary to cope with the stress. If you have no reason to believe your situation will improve, give yourself permission to leave your job. Many nurses are drawn to their profession because of their gifts and inner needs to care for others. Although these qualities are admirable and serve others well, they do not always serve the caretaker well. Resigning a position does not mean you are a failure. It could be a way to take control of your life and afford yourself the type of care and attention you are so good at giving to others.

In most instances, your work environment will be manageable and you will be able to support yourself and your staff. Below are recommendations for supporting yourself.

Wilson[7] recommends the following tips for nurses dealing with the stress of their profession. These tips apply to staff nurses as well as to nurse managers.

TIPS TO SUPPORT YOURSELF

✔ Develop a "can do" attitude. Consider the problems you *can* solve and focus on these, rather than all the problems you *can not* solve. These successes will help you feel capable, stronger, and more able to take on the next problem.

✔ Become more assertive. Feeling powerless in your relationships is a great source of job stress. Learn constructive ways to solve problems and communicate effectively with others—not aggressively, but calmly, directly, and with respect for yourself and others. Take a class or workshop in communications or assertiveness.

✔ Make overwhelming tasks manageable. Break down big tasks into their component parts. Then concentrate on completing each part. At the beginning of the day, instead of feeling powerless in the face of the next 8 to 10 hours of work, prioritize and write down your tasks for the next 30 minutes, 2 hours, 4 hours, and so on. Then take them a step at a time.

✔ Manage your time better. Combine tasks when you can. If you have to make a call, before you pick up the phone, consider if you have other matters to discuss with the same person or department. If you take a patient admission history, write it directly onto the form. Do not write it on scratch paper and copy it later onto the form. Learn to delegate when appropriate. Do not think you have to do *everything*. Learn what you must do to take care of yourself and what can be expected of others.

✔ Accept your failures, and do not take yourself so seriously. When you fail, look at what went wrong and why, and consider whether you could have done something differently. Learn from your mistakes and resolve to put this learning to use. Accept that you are human and that you will make mistakes. Learn to laugh at yourself sometimes and appreciate the good things around you.

✔ Nurture each other. Use your caretaking skills with one another. Cultivate friendships with people you trust.

✔ Nurture yourself. Learn to relax, listen to your body's needs for caretaking, exercise, and do something fun for yourself at least once a week.

More Tips for Taking Care of Yourself

The following are other ways to support yourself and alleviate the effects of routine stress on a short-term and long-term basis. Work to stop a molehill of stress from building to a mountain. Many of these suggestions also could be helpful for your staff. We saved the best lists for last.

SHORT-TERM STRESS: TIPS IF YOU ARE FEELING TENSE AT WORK

✔ Ask a coworker to relieve you for a few moments so you can adjust your thinking and put things in perspective.

✔ Take a few minutes to sit down, take some deep breaths, and relax.

✔ Step away from the work environment and stretch your arms and legs, touch your toes, and open and close your fists to release tension.

✔ Take a moment to think of an enjoyable time you had with a friend or family member. Let yourself smile.

✔ Take a moment to visualize yourself as a relaxed, capable individual who *can* solve problems.

✔ Take a few minutes to consult with a peer, ventilate, and perhaps get a different perspective.

✔ Make up your mind that the stressful situation at hand will not get the better of you.

LONG-TERM STRESS: TIPS FOR THE REST OF YOUR LIFE

✔ Take time to "smell the roses" everyday. Do something just for you, no matter how small. Watch a favorite television program, talk to a friend on the phone, take a walk, give yourself a pedicure, or curl up in bed an hour early and catch up on your reading.

✔ Get a manicure, facial, or a new haircut.

✔ Get regular physical exercise, such as walking, jogging, swimming, or gardening.

✔ Eat healthful foods. Limit caffeine and alcoholic beverages.

✔ Ventilate tension from work by talking for 5 or 10 minutes to a sympathetic listener—a spouse, friend, coworker. Talk in general terms—"Two people died today," or "We had to work short today." Avoid detailed discussions or blow-by-blow accounts of your day, which only serve to make you relive the stress a second time, instead of relieving it. The object is simply to feel the support of someone who cares about you.

✔ Learn to meditate. Meditation is a good way to focus yourself and to relax. Fifteen to thirty minutes of meditation in the morning or evening will go a long way toward helping you keep perspective for the rest of your day.

✔ Build your relationships with your peer group. Sharing concerns, considering solutions to routine problems, and enjoying one another's company all are good ways to give and receive support.

✔ Schedule regular vacations, usually at 3-month or 4-month intervals. In the interim, a 3-day weekend can provide a great deal of relaxation.

✔ Leave work at work. Plan so that you are not taking home work on a regular basis.

✔ Cultivate outside interests that are unrelated to your work. Include individuals who are not in the health care field in your circle of friends.

✔ Ask your supervisor to set up time with you to brainstorm solutions to particularly stressful situations.

✔ Stay tuned to the stress level of your staff. The more quickly you address their stress, the less likely serious problems will develop.

✔ Participate in professional development, quality control, or other committees in your work setting. This involvement will help you become more familiar with your institution, help you to network, provide different perspectives on situations and problems in your job, and give you exposure for recognition for your good ideas and work.

✔ Be active in your professional organizations. Through this participation, you will learn nursing and management skills, as well as networking and strengthening peer relationships. As a result, you will feel stronger, smarter, and less stressed.

✔ Be realistic about the problems on your job. Not every problem is your responsibility, and you can not solve the world's problems. Take responsibility for only those problems which are yours.

✔ Have realistic expectations of others. Eliminate the stress of being frustrated by inconsequential shortcomings of others.

✔ Keep a positive attitude. Bad attitudes are contagious and breed additional stress.

✔ Address and correct mistakes. Then forgive yourself and others for making mistakes.

SUMMARY

This chapter reviewed stress in the nursing workplace and how it can manifest itself, stress coping mechanisms, and signs of unmanaged stress. Examples of serious staff problems and recommended actions were discussed. Also, the unmanageable environment was explored, as were points on how to recognize this "no-win" situation.

Many suggestions were made about supporting yourself and your staff. Undoubtedly you can think of additional ways—ways that apply specifically to you or to your staff.

No single reference, person, or resource contains all the answers to a given situation or problem. Talk to your supervisor and your peers. Read professional journals. Continue your efforts to seek information and develop your own solutions to take care of yourself and your staff. The return on your investment will be great.

REFERENCES

1. Nicholson L: Stress management in nursing, *Nurs Manage* 21(4):53, 1990.
2. Foxall MJ, et al: A comparison of frequency and sources of nursing job stress perceived by intensive care, hospice and medical-surgical nurses, *J Adv Nurs* 15(5):577, 1990.
3. Lees S, Ellis N: The design of a stress-management programme for nursing personnel, *J Adv Nurs* 15:946, 1990.
4. Simms L, et al: Breaking the burn-out barrier: resurrecting work excitement in nursing," *Nurs Economics* 8(3):185, 1990.
5. Robinson JA, Lewis DJ: Coping with ICU work-related stressors: a study, *Crit Care Nurse* 10(5):86, 1990.
6. Breakwell GM: Are you stressed out?, *Am J Nurs*, 90(8):31, 1990. Article abstracted from Breakwell GM: *Facing physical violence*, first published in London, 1990, The British Psychological Society in association with Routledge Ltd, and 1990, New York, Chapman & Hall.
7. Wilson LK: High-gear nursing: how it can run you down and what you can do about it, *Nursing '89* 19(12):81, 1989.
8. Bissell L, Jones D: The alcoholic nurse, *Nurs Outlook* 29:96, 1981.
9. Selbach KH: Chemical dependency in nursing, *AORN J* 52(3):531, 1990.
10. Albrecht TL, Halsey J: Supporting the staff nurse under stress, *Nurs Manage* 22(7):60, July, 1991.
11. Smith LB: Humor relations for nurse managers, *Nurs Manage* 21(5): 86, 1990.

CHAPTER 11

When Bad Things Happen to Good Managers

T. M. Marrelli

Certain problems commonly faced in management are unpleasant or difficult for many managers. Hopefully you will not experience many of them. However, they do occur and should be addressed. These problems can be as simple as feeling vulnerable during the transition from nurse to manager and wanting to stay in the former role. You must put these problems into perspective. Although they alone usually are not good reasons for leaving a position that you otherwise would enjoy, they can make you feel like leaving. Some of the most common problems faced by new managers are discussed in this chapter.

SPECIAL PROBLEMS
When You Are Promoted And Your Friend Is Not

When you are chosen for a management position, a friend or close colleague who also applied for the position may feel hurt, disappointed, or resentful. Your friend's reaction may, in turn, make you feel sad, disappointed, or even guilty. These feelings can be incredibly uncomfortable and usually do not go away overnight. You must remember that you are now the manager and were chosen over your friend for a reason, although you probably should not verbalize this to your friend. In addition, no matter how happy your friend may appear for you, hurt feelings will probably arise. You cannot pretend that the relationship has not changed; it has by the nature of the hierarchy in the workplace. The change can be particularly difficult if you have been long-term peers and have experienced parallel careers and a close friendship. Although your goal may be to stay close friends, this may be difficult. It depends on you and your friend. The new manager must realize that favorites or perceived favorites cannot exist on a cohesive team. Therefore you can do the following to ease the transition.

TIPS ON DEALING WITH A CLOSE FRIEND AFTER YOUR PROMOTION

✔ Do not apologize even if you feel somewhat guilty about receiving the promotion.

✔ Do not give your friend favorable treatment. Your guilt may cause you to want to "protect" your friend, which will cause problems with other staff members.

✔ Try to ignore the situation if your friend teases you verbally about the position (e.g., referring to you as the big honcho). However, you will have to set limits on this behavior if it continues.

✔ You can try to maintain your social relationship, but you must accept that it will change. Obviously, your social relationship must be kept outside the work setting. Sometimes the relationship will deteriorate, and you may have to accept this loss.

✔ Work on achieving mutual respect. Bringing professional behaviors and effective interpersonal skills to these uncomfortable situations can help. The effort expended to maintain the friendship can be draining, and the transition period can be disheartening for new managers.

✔ Give this process time. Your friend may need space initially while getting used to the change. Eventually you and your friend may be able to resume the friendship.

✔ Discuss with other nurse managers how they have addressed and solved this problem. Such support can be beneficial to you in this uncomfortable situation.

Discomfort in an Unfamiliar Environment

Because hospitals and health care settings must now be more financially oriented to thrive and even survive, some changes are being felt in the workplace. The new nurse manager can be overwhelmed by the red tape, politics, and sabotage that sometimes occur. To help you adjust, the following tips can help.

TIPS ON ADJUSTING TO A NEW ENVIRONMENT

✔ Talk to trusted peer nurse managers on an ongoing basis.

✔ Introduce yourself to everyone you can. Ask people to lunch or to tell you about their role in the organization. People love to talk about themselves and their accomplishments, and these meetings can give you the needed insight into the corporate culture that you would not find on the organizational chart or in the recruitment brochure.

✔ Watch how people communicate with each other (formal, informal, memos) and observe nuances that are unique to your work setting.

✔ Rely on both the grapevine and feedback. Unfortunately, in some environments, there is poor communication from the top levels to the ranks below. If you are in this type of environment, the grapevine may often provide more information than do formal communications.

✔ Try to remain objective. If your current setting operates differently from the last setting you worked in, give your new organization time to demonstrate how it works before judging and trying to implement major changes.

Firing or Letting Go of a Staff Member

Probably no management process is as difficult to be involved in as firing a staff member. This process can be especially challenging for new managers. When there are serious and ongoing problems with a staff member, discuss the situation with both your immediate supervisor and the HR manager. You should not attempt to handle this process without adequate support, particularly if the staff member's problems precede your tenure. For a more in-depth discussion of firing, please refer to Chapter 3.

Times of High Stress or Anxiety

Maclaren said, "What does anxiety do? It does not empty tomorrow of its sorrow; rather it empties today of its strength" (Jan Maclaren, 1920). As nurses, we all know the symptoms of anxiety and stress. Probably few, if any, management positions exist in which stress is not a hallmark of daily life. You must remember that some stress is good and that the way you view your relationship to stress can help you master it. You must take steps to control stress or channel it into productive activities.

You can use the uncomfortable feelings stress creates as catalysts for needed change and to learn new or more effective behaviors. Yet, when you are stressed, you may not feel like doing anything that affects or solves the problem. At these times, you may want to meet with peers or other appropriate staff members such as the social worker or the psychiatric liaison nurse. Some facilities provide nurse managers with counseling to assist them through change and crisis and also to help them support their own staff. J.L. Casey, a nurse, said the following about this positive process.

Through the counseling sessions, the clinician helped me to understand group dynamics and to learn how to support the staff effectively in times of stress or change. Also, she enabled me to gain an awareness of my own personal management style and of how others react to me. Indeed, the clinician's support has alleviated much of the stress of my new job. She has given me the courage to meet new challenges and to continue to grow and develop both professionally and personally.[1]

Please refer to Chapter 10 for an in-depth discussion on stress and stress management.

Unfulfilled Promises by Management

It can be disheartening when your supervisor makes promises that are not kept. This is why many employment counselors suggest obtaining a written job offer with all details specified before accepting a position. Unfulfilled promises can also occur with bonuses, promotions, or other aspects of your employment. Broken promises erode trust and can be damaging to morale and productivity. It is best to avoid making promises, either actual or implied, to your staff unless you are certain that you can fulfill the promises.

Unreasonable or Bad Managers

"In a recent study of 73 managers conducted by the University of Southern California, nearly 75% of the participants reported having had difficulty with a superior. Moreover, bad-boss behavior appears to be on the rise."[2] It is hoped that you never work for someone who expects more every day when you have no hope of getting the staff or other resources needed to do the tasks. The continual feeling that you can never do enough can lead to burnout. The successful nurse manager must set limits and know what can be accomplished effectively and realistically in what time frames and with what resources. Network with your peers to validate your perceptions. You may find that you are not alone and that they may have developed coping skills to assist them in remaining fairly content in their positions. Their advice and insight may help you to cope with your situation.

Little or No Management Training

Perhaps your "management training" consisted of the regular staff nurse orientation accompanied by a videotape on assertive behavior and a 2-hour session on HR management! Then you were left to sink or swim. This is a problem. To successfully make the transition to management and function as an effective manager, the new nurse manager should receive structured training related to management issues, concepts, skills, and techniques. If you do not feel that you received the orientation you need, talk to your supervisor about your specific needs. Do not be embarrassed—you are entitled to an orientation commensurate with your responsibilities. To supplement formal educational offerings, you can also offer to lead a peer nurse manager workshop and have the new group define the topics on which orientation is needed. Responsibility for running these meetings can be rotated among the members. It might be helpful to invite and involve your facility's staff development coordinator. Reading the numerous books and journals available can also help you develop your management expertise. Educational offerings such as workshops, courses, and conferences can further enhance your understanding and mastery of management. Resources for Further Professional Development, located at the end of the book, may be helpful in facilitating development of your management expertise.

Following in the Footsteps of Multiple and Short-Term Managers

When you inherit staff members who have been through a lot of change, problems abound. Initially, it may be best to observe before making changes of your own. In addition, the staff may feel you will be another short-term manager and may be skeptical. Considering the numerous changes, the setting may need some structure. One way to provide structure is to improve the organization of the unit. Look at your office and talk to peer nurse managers to determine which files are truly needed. Use aids such as accordion binders or a scheduling board to help you feel more organized. The simple acts of organizing the mess may help you and your staff feel less overwhelmed. Get vertical files, bookcases, and whatever else is needed to gain some control over your new environment. Remember and practice organizational skills. Integrating these skills into your daily work life will result in the following:

1. A sense of accomplishment
2. A feeling of control over your space
3. More time to do the task at hand; namely managing the unit
4. Demonstrating organization for your staff

It may take your staff time to believe that you will be the manager for an extended period. Sometimes such frequent changes create strong and effective staff members because they have functioned as the leaders for their unit throughout the gaps and turnover of managers. This staff may also have had to adjust to very different management styles and expectations over time and knows what works best for the unit. Because of these factors, the staff members can be knowledgeable resources about their unit. They may have good ideas about the stability and direction needed on the unit and contribute positively to these goals. Encourage staff members to share their ideas. For a more in-depth discussion on organizational skills, see Chapter 6.

Your Supervisor's Negative Evaluation of You

Performance evaluations can be difficult for both the evaluator and the employee being evaluated. If your supervisor gives you a poor or average evaluation, you must, with her help, determine the cause or causes. Try to be objective and put yourself in the evaluator's position. Does your supervisor feel uninformed? Are you generally late with work projects? Are you loyal? Do you follow through when your supervisor delegates work to you? Does your supervisor feel respected by you?

Sometimes it is hard to remember that your supervisor is your supervisor and, as such, must be considered correct. If you are surprised by your supervisor's negative evaluation, you can ask for additional feedback on an ongoing basis to gauge your progress. Ask what specific behaviors are problems and how you can demonstrate improvement to your supervisor. If you are in a new position, it is important to remember that you probably will not perform exceptionally from the start. Stress your interest in learning and improving and ask for your supervisor's help.

A disappointing performance evaluation can be particularly frustrating in those instances where the supervisor promoted you into the position or recruited you for the job. You may feel misled or even betrayed. If you feel that you did not receive an adequate management orientation, you may wish to request additional training. Look objectively at your job description and objectively demonstrate, in writing if need be, the ways you feel you meet the position standards. Whatever you do, especially in the current economic climate, do not tell your supervisor that she is wrong. Other mistakes to avoid are blaming others and constantly complaining (especially about issues over which your supervisor has no control).

Also, consider how your supervisor deals with other nurse managers she supervises. If she frequently praises a peer nurse manager, observe what your peer does differently or better than you. Perhaps you have not gained recognition for your accomplishments. We all would like to believe that good work gets recognized and reinforced, but, in reality, sometimes the squeaky wheel gets the attention. In this case, the squeaky wheel also gets the positive strokes and evaluations. Some people have a knack for pointing out to their supervisors just what they are doing that is wonderful, helps the organization look good, and most importantly, makes the supervisor look great. No one likes to be self congratulatory, but sometimes you may need to bring your achievements to your supervisor's attention.

When You Do Not Get the Recognition You Deserve

The questions that follow may help you identify whether you are getting the recognition you deserve. Your supervisor may not know what you are doing, and it may appear that the work you are accomplishing is minimal. This situation particularly can be seen in some settings where there are bonuses. Workers who toot their own horns and come out ahead are not necessarily better workers; they may simply be better at public relations and at communicating to their managers what the managers want and need to hear.

The following questions can help you determine if you are doing your part to receive the recognition you deserve.

DOING YOUR PART TO RECEIVE RECOGNITION

✔ Do people at different levels of the organization know who you are?

✔ Do you volunteer for assignments or opportunities to increase your visibility?

✔ Do you routinely tell your supervisor about your accomplishments?

✔ Sometimes we may be hassled or nervous when we meet with our supervisors, and we may neglect to refer to our accomplishments. Try to make it a point to always have three accomplishments to tell your supervisor about at the onset of your meetings. The supervisor wants to see objective results too, so in turn your boss's boss may hear those same items. This positive action reflects on your boss and can only help you.

✔ Do you share your unit's accomplishments with your staff and encourage them to share their individual accomplishments with you?

✔ Have your staff enumerate three accomplishments every week that you can then present to your supervisor. It will help your staff feel a part of the team. In addition, the knowledge that you share this information with your boss will increase their feeling that you are all working together.

WHEN YOU IDENTIFY THE NEED FOR A CHANGE IN YOUR JOB

Occasionally, your work situation may be so uncomfortable that you want to leave your position. When you are unhappy at work, you must try to determine specifically why you feel that way. Such information will help you identify the actions you need to take to improve the situation. All jobs have inherent pros and cons. The important issue is that the position meets your unique needs. The decision to leave is usually reached when all actions taken fail. Many skills are available to try to affect a negative work situation.

Problem solving, conflict resolution, and other avenues toward finding solutions should be attempted when possible. However, note that sometimes, even when your job is fulfilling, it simply may be time for a change. At some point, people consider changing careers entirely. Knowing when to leave can sometimes result from intuition and honest discussions with trusted friends or colleagues.

Many businesses will welcome an RN on their staff's roster. Nurses have many job opportunities that tie together health interests and other activities. Some of these include health care–related sales such as computers, medical equipment, or supplies; programs for the aging; nursing staffing companies; medicolegal consulting; research; health or hospital administration; liaison between facilities; teaching; insurance utilization review; case management services; private practice; lobbying; and occupational health and wellness programs. For an in-depth discussion about other opportunities and marketing yourself and your skills, refer to Chapter 13, which specifies steps that may help you find the right position or identify the next professional stage in your career.

THE BOTTOM LINE

"'It was much pleasanter at home, thought poor Alice, when one wasn't always growing larger and smaller, and being ordered around by mice and rabbits. I almost wish I hadn't gone down that rabbit hole . . . !'

The thoughts and experiences of Lewis Carroll's Alice are an eloquent parallel to those of nurses in middle management roles. Many wish to go 'home' to bedside nursing, where one is not accountable to, and responsible for, everyone above and below (all those mice and rabbits!), besides being responsible for quality patient care. The step into management, be it prompted by curiosity, ambition, or a desire to contribute, can mimic Alice's dreamlike fall down the rabbit hole, complete with changes in size and form, and encounters with all kinds of mysterious characters."[3] Determine if your current position has the critical elements needed to make you happy and effectively use your special skills and abilities. It is important that you spend some time considering those aspects of the position which are satisfying as well as those which are not. Weighing these criteria will assist you in deciding whether to move on. This is also the time to reflect on your perception of problems. Those who frame problems as challenges and find solutions seem to enjoy their work more. In addition, although every setting has different problems, some types of problems are inherent in management and may follow you regardless of the setting in which you work.

SUMMARY

Problems appear in many facets of our worklives. It is important to realize and sometimes remind ourselves that we are not alone. The good point about addressing problems is that once we problem-solve or identify the action needed for resolution, we have one less to address. In addition, some problems, after initially being addressed, serve as precedents for our way of effectively handling similar problems. With these facts in mind, problem-solving becomes easier. For example, human relation problems are varied and can be addressed in many ways. However, your facility policy manuals and your supervisor are resources for guidance or responses needed during the period of transition to experienced nurse manager. Your peer nurse managers can be a source of support and of information about "how do you handle" issues. A peer manager meeting on problem solving and conflict resolution may be a particularly effective method of increasing your comfort level, obtaining support, and increasing your job knowledge.

We learn from our experiences, and the problems become easier to solve with time and experience. Addressing the problems is what is important. We cannot have all the right answers all the time. There are resources in your chain of command to help you during this time, and it is important that you use them when needed. You must realize that being a manager is a continual growth process. This process can be facilitated through the reading of professional books or journals and participating in workshops or attending courses.

In your capacity as manager, you are the role model for your staff. This cyclical process of training members of your staff through delegation, empowerment, and their assumption of accountability develops their skills to professionally grow and perhaps become managers themselves.

REFERENCES

1. Casey JL: Counseling nurse managers, *Nurs Manage* 20(9):53, September, 1989.
2. Lopez JA: The boss from hell, *Working Woman* page 69, December, 1991.
3. Boll ML: Middle management in nursing, *Nurs Manage* 21(2):54, 1990.

The Nurse Manager in Homecare and Hospice

T.M. Marrelli

HOW HOMECARE IS UNIQUE

Homecare itself is different for many reasons. The reasons center primarily around the fact that health care providers are guests in their client's homes. Unlike the inpatient setting, visiting hours are not set and patients have control over their environment and numerous other choices within their homes, including their clothing, food, visitors, and lifestyle. The care provider must be the one to adjust whenever accommodation is necessary. This customer-oriented or service-driven philosophy is what makes the home setting so different from other clinical environments. To support this structure, we need to see how the nurses who make visits or provide care at home bring special skills to the homecare position. This is not to say that nurses in inpatient areas do not have some or even all of these traits. Rather, this chapter concerns the attributes that must be developed by effective homecare managers for professional nurses to remain in homecare and addresses the specifics of homecare management that are not integrated into the other chapters.

HOMECARE AND HOSPICE CONSIDERATIONS

The multifaceted administrative and clinical operations that must be maintained to provide patient care are the core of the homecare manager's responsibilities. Be aware that all the chapters, for example, Chapter 7, "Budgeting Basics," and Chapter 10, "Taking Care of You and Your Staff," are relevant to homecare managers. Stress management skills are needed by all managers, and the budgeting discussions are particularly relevant in homecare. In fact, one example of productivity in the budgeting chapter is a home health agency (HHA) example.

The management skills needed in home health and hospice are many and varied. They range from effective recruiting and hiring of skilled and interpersonally effective clinicians to the ongoing duties needed to achieve timely and correct billing submissions. Although the term *homecare* is used throughout this discussion, this discussion is germane to all care provided primarily in the patient's home. Therefore this information is also relevant for hospice care or other special programs that emphasize providing care at home. Because many hospices are affiliated or otherwise associated with a homecare agency, the term *homecare* is used generically for ease of discussion. *Homecare* is also used in this chapter for all homecare programs, including HHAs. Regardless of the type of care program provided at home, the manager's duties and responsibilities are directed toward the maintenance of effective daily operations to provide high-quality patient care.

This chapter is organized with an overview of the hallmarks that make up the professional practice of homecare, the regulatory aspects and requirements, and patient care considerations. The overview includes important issues such as how patient/nurse assignments are made, the practice models used, automated systems, the documentation requirements, and the unique billing/administrative functions that the manager must direct on a daily basis. A homecare and hospice resource guide is located at the end of this book for your information and for continued professional growth.

HOW HOMECARE MANAGEMENT IS UNIQUE

You were probably promoted from being a staff homecare nurse to being a manager because of your clinical competence, expertise, and other valued skills. However, in addition, the new manager in homecare must be willing to achieve or possess the following skills and knowledge:

- An indepth knowledge of the current regulatory environment, including the Medicare Conditions of Participation (COPs) and state surveyor interpretations for compliance with them, and the state Certificate of Need (CON), and Licensure laws, where applicable. Also, the manager must know the status (and source) of accreditation and the complex multifaceted "rules" that are synonymous with homecare, including the HHA Health Insurance Manual (HIM-11), the specific provisions for coverage, and the documentation requirements in the HIM-11.

- Knowledge of the billing procedures and rules that dictate the administrative structures and processes necessary to support timely and effective billing. The administrative skills needed to orchestrate the many steps that must occur require flexibility. A structure that moves the process forward regardless of staffing problems or other operational problems is demanded. This is part of being the manager and being accountable for the fiscal health of the HHA. Please refer to Chapter 6 for an indepth discussion about effective time management and productivity.

- A repertoire of service-driven and patient-oriented interpersonal skills. Unlike many inpatient facilities, where the structure defines the services, in homecare, because the patient is at home, the patient's needs are the criteria that drive the program. These skills are also highly valued in the manager's role in public relations or community liaison activities, which are a daily part of effective homecare operations.

- The experience base and knowledge to successfully and credibly deal with complex situations that may be addressed exclusively over the phone and through documentation. In the inpatient setting, the nurses are down the hall or closer. In homecare, your delegation, communication, or follow-up interventions are with staff members who may be four counties away or even across the state line. This is why there is such as emphasis on continuous quality improvement in homecare, including the ongoing and systematic process of comparing patient episodes of care by like diagnoses or other similar factors affecting patient outcomes.

- Possession of an incredible attention to detail. This is especially true in the important daily operations of (1) billing and (2) documentation. Because these two factors go hand in hand, they are equally important. An HHA manager that does not send bills or bills incorrectly is jeopardizing the viability of the organization. In addition, the HHA that does not have the necessary documentation to support the bills not only faces problems from a risk-management standpoint, but also from the payor's view. The payor may view this situation as overutilization, a gray zone that may indicate abuse or even fraud. The documentation in billing and the clinical records must be correct for any audit trail.

HOW HOMECARE NURSES ARE UNIQUE

In the accompanying box are listed some of the unique characteristics of nurses and the homecare setting. Obviously, the management skills needed for success in homecare are many and varied. They range from the effective hiring of skilled and interpersonally strong clinicians to the ongoing orchestration of duties to achieve timely billing submissions.

UNIQUE CHARACTERISTICS

1. The staff must be flexible. It is homecare staff members who must bend or renegotiate, not the patient, as members are guests in their home. This usually includes visit times but can include aspects of the plan of care as well.
2. The staff member must not mind driving, even in inclement weather, have a good sense of direction, and be willing to take risks (i.e., get lost).
3. The staff members assume responsibility for the patient and the patient's plan of care. True primary nursing or case management occurs in homecare. From the initial assessment visit, through to identifying and using appropriate nursing diagnoses, the nurse in homecare assumes the planning and follow-through of care. Possibly only one or maybe a limited number of team members are involved in the care, depending on the patient's needs. These team members directly affect the care and see the results of care provided. Because of this, the outcomes may be more directly attributable to care rendered. This total patient management function, with its associated prioritizing and complex decision-making, renders this field unique. Note that in practice, the simple, positive patient and family outcomes and feedback are where many homecare nurses receive a great deal of personal and job satisfaction. Because of this factor, this feedback also needs to be highly valued by all members of the management team.
4. Staff members must be generalists and specialists. This means that, although clinically the RNs may be able to competently and proficiently handle a wide range of patients and clinical problems, they usually have an area of expertise that can be called on for specialized clinical problems, orientation of new staff, or as a resource for information.
5. The staff must be autonomous and able to function in a nonstructured atmosphere.
6. The staff must have effective time management skills regarding both visits scheduled and documentation/administrative duties required. The amount of detail management that must be mastered is key to long-term success for many nurses in homecare. For example, the tracking of recertifications, 486 generation and visit schedules demand nurses who are detail oriented and even value that detail. In addition, plans made between the nurse and patient must be followed up in actuality and on paper.

Continued.

UNIQUE CHARACTERISTICS—cont'd

7. The staff must be open and accepting of people's unique and chosen lifestyles and the associated effects on their health. Judgements about lifestyle, the presence or absence of family support, and the choices patients make with which nurses do not agree must be diplomatically and carefully voiced when appropriate.
8. The staff must like to interact with patients and their families and caregivers. This teaching or consulting role also brings job satisfaction to nurses in home health.
9. The staff must be aware that a constant balance exists between the clinical and administrative demands and that each are equally important, but in different ways and for different reasons.
10. The staff must be aware that successful mastery of time management and delegation skills are essential to effective daily operations.

The nurses who choose homecare must be able to function somewhat autonomously. Consider the inpatient ICU nurse who goes into homecare thinking it will be "less stressful" and finds the culture so different, that she cannot successfully make the transition to independent and successful homecare nursing. With this in mind, plan orientation periods with the goal of the participant's having long-term success in the role. We know change is difficult, and the homecare nurse culture and setting is different from the structure and on-site comraderie, supervision, and peer consultation available from the structure of a facility. Similarly, your orientation as a new manager must be effective for you to competently and efficiently carry out your new management responsibilities.

THE NEW MANAGER'S ORIENTATION TO HOMECARE

There are too many stories of homecare managers who get no orientation and not surprisingly get burnt out or disillusioned and leave their position, homecare, or even nursing. Do not let this "revolving door" phenomena happen to you. All managers are entitled to an appropriate orientation period. No matter how understaffed the administrator says the agency is, protect yourself from being put in that position from the start. Try to define or address your orientation, including time span and content, before accepting the position. The following discussion addresses what details your orientation should include.

WHAT YOUR ORIENTATION SHOULD ENTAIL

The items in the accompanying box are the *minimal* topics that can be considered to provide an effective orientation to homecare. Obviously, if you have been in homecare for some time, some of these may not be appropriate or needed, but all managers should have these "hallmarks" of homecare as a base of information. In addition, these items will give you information about the HHA's internal operations.

HALLMARKS OF ORIENTATION

1. The HHA orientation manual.
2. The conditions of participation.
3. The HHA's continuous quality improvement program. The HHA should share their last quarterly or last few quarterly report(s). This will help you to follow-up on areas that needed improvement before your tenure began. If no report exists or "one was not done last quarter," this could indicate why they need your skills. Obviously, this can be a good or a bad sign!
4. The HIM-11,[1] especially Transmittal 222, the HHA Coverage Requirements section.
5. The clinical policy and procedure manuals.
6. The human resource policy manual, including position descriptions.
7. Organizational chart and current staffing needs. This includes who you report to and who has true (not just on paper) responsibilities for specific areas.
8. The staff education and inservice training log.
9. An overview of the medical records and documentation system.
10. An overview of the clinical/billing/administrative automated system information, where applicable.
11. A schematic diagram of the paper flow process from patient intake/admission to billing and discharge.
12. The HHA's fiscal statements and accounts pending, and the most recent cost reports, where appropriate.
13. The caseload of the previous months/year.
14. The HHA's annual report.
15. Their interest in or their actual accreditation status.
16. The HHA's strategic plan.
17. Community linkage and involvement.
18. The HHA's denial rate.
19. The HHA's participation in state and national industry organizations.
20. Other information as needed.

Orienting a new manager should take at least as long as it does for a new clinical nurse in homecare. Much of the above information is also appropriate (except financial) for the new nurse in homecare. Remember, the more managers communicate the program's goals or visions, the more staff members feel a part of the team and are thereby more effective.

It goes without saying that your staff members cannot be held accountable for what they do not or could not know if they did not get an effective orientation. With this in mind, and from your perspective as the risk manager and person in charge of CQI, adequately train your homecare nursing staff. Like you, their manager, they need to know the cornerstones of information about homecare. These should **always** include such basic topics as home visits and what they entail, including buddying with an experienced, positive role model nurse; visit utilization; orientation to the forms used; infection control; and coverage and associated documentation requirements of homecare services and CQI processes. The manager cannot be effective if she does not know the program, the key players, and the expected performance goals. Similarly, it is difficult and usually unfair to hold staff members accountable for information of which they were unaware. Be a prudent manager: orient your team effectively.

IF YOU HAVE TO NEGOTIATE FOR AN ORIENTATION

If you are in the unfortunate position of bargaining for an adequate orientation, there is a problem. Most professional nurses want to be affiliated with high-quality programs. However, believing that all homecare programs are functioning at the same (high-quality) level would be naive. There may be instances when your supervisor uses the word "quality," but that same supervisor's actions concern you. Trust your nursing knowledge and experience. Look to the professional standards of care for guidance and more information.

If you are always needing information to do your job, if you cannot do your job effectively because of no orientation or support, or if you are a manager in "title" but are continually in the field seeing patients because of incredible turnover, you are experiencing problems that may not be resolved by your management. Note that you cannot be expected to be in the community making visits and also be in the office supervising agency operations. This is a prescription for failure in any busy HHA setting. Clinical and administrative demands are so different that to attempt both is ineffective.

Another uncomfortable position that a manager can be involved in entails the admission of patients clearly needing homecare services and not having the personnel resources available to provide them. For example, the admitting nurse identifies appropriately a patient's need for skilled intermittent nursing service and, because of extensive personal care needs, frequent home health aide visits. Your agency does not have the aides (or the speech/language pathologists or the physical or occupational therapists) to adequately meet the patient's care needs. When possible, admit patients where their care needs can be safely and adequately met. It is most unfortunate, and certainly not fair to the patients or their family members, if patients do not receive the services they clearly need because of the HHA's administrative problems. The necessity of demonstrating quality in patient care cannot be underestimated. As competition continues, as more programs receive accreditation, and as HHA licensure increases throughout the country, HHAs appear more uniform. However, as inpatient days of care continue to be shortened, and HHAs to appear alike, only those HHAs which are truly responsive to patients and where patients perceive they received high-quality care will survive.

QUALITY IN OPERATIONS

Much discussion is underway now about accreditation in homecare. Both the NLN and the JCAHO accredit homecare programs of all auspices. The design and implementation of a quality assurance program in your agency must meet your agency's unique clinical focuses. Many agencies incorporate operational aspects into their CQI program. Often it encompasses tracking patients and patient information regarding episodes of hospital readmissions within 31 days, complaint trends, ongoing clinical record reviews, infection surveillance and rates, and focused studies. It may also includes patient, physician, and referral source satisfaction surveys. The manager in homecare must be on the HHA's CQI committee. In addition, the homecare nurses need to have a voice in operations.

The educational preparation and clinical knowledge and experience of the homecare nurse can be another measure of quality. A new certification in homecare is being offered by the American Nurses' Credentialing Center. This new specialty certification is a way to help ensure that nurses in homecare know and practice within standard quality parameters.

The nursing care delivery system model used in the HHA can also affect the quality of the care provided by affecting patient outcomes. For an in-depth discussion on quality, please refer to Chapter 9, "Quality Assessment and Improvement."

MODELS OF NURSING CARE DELIVERY SYSTEMS IN HOMECARE

Various models in homecare describe how care is delivered to HHA patients. Primary nursing through assignment of client/patient care managers (or case managers in some settings) is model frequently seen in homecare. We all recognize that continuity through primary nursing care models promotes professional accountability and increased effectiveness in communications and outcomes. The manager's knowledge of each staff member's preparation, experience, and capabilities promotes the fullest use of skills and provides a basis for continued growth.

Regardless of the model used, assigning a nurse who has the overall responsibility for implementing and evaluating the ordered plan of care is a key to positive patient outcomes. The purpose of assigning one nurse to this responsibility is to help ensure the quality of the care by providing a mechanism for consistent rapport and communications for the patient and his caregivers. Clearly, this is not to say that additional nursing staff such as "associate nurses" are not also involved in the care of the patient. In fact, involving another nurse can be helpful. For example, a nurse specialist, such as an enterostomal therapist, could consult on appropriate cases, thus assuring quality while providing patient care in a consultative role. Assigning homecare nurses to patients, in keeping with your organizational philosophy, also supports nursing care assignments that are directed toward meeting the specific physical, psychologic, social, and other defined needs of each patient.

This assignment is most effectively accomplished by the nurse manager evaluating the projected identified needs of patients as soon as possible after the referral process has occurred. The effective manager accomplishes this by gathering all the available and pertinent information about the patient and his care needs. The manager then assesses the availability of RN resources. This includes the number of staff members and their clinical expertise, educational preparation, experience, and demonstrated capabilities. Matching of patients and nurses is sometimes referred to as "skill matching" or "care matching." In addition, the manager considers the individual preferences of staff members while evaluating the complexity or extent of patient needs. Consideration for the preferences of nursing staff members needs to be kept in mind and valued, as this positively influences the morale of the group.

Information concerning preferences needs to be acquired in a systematic way, such as regular individual staff meetings with the manager, to ensure all staff members are given equal consideration. The assignment process is also made with the primary nurse's current patient caseload in mind. Geographic location and equitable work distribution are two additional factors to consider. In addition, matching assignments to the abilities and growth potential of the professional staff member enhances the quality of care, is cost effective, increases productivity, and promotes staff member satisfaction. Effective managers work with their staff to assist them, when possible, in understanding the rationale of assignments.

Depending on your chosen nursing model, the delegation of responsibility for planning, supervising, and evaluating the total nursing care of the patient occurs when the patient is assigned to the primary nurse.

Communications with your staff on an ongoing basis are the key to a successful operation where all efforts are directed toward common goals. Though the bulk of daily communications with your clinical staff will be over the phone, it is important that you see your staff on a regular basis. The following box addresses the important role of staff meetings in homecare and hospice.

THE IMPORTANCE OF STAFF MEETINGS IN HOMECARE AND HOSPICE

The importance of regularly scheduled staff meetings in the homecare or hospice office cannot be understated. Because the very nature and definition of the care provision is external, the staff members need to be and feel a part of the group. Staff meetings assist in meeting both the staff and manager's goals. Though you may define the agenda, ask your staff members for issues or concerns they want addressed and incorporate the items whenever possible. Make the staff meetings and their agenda items and ensuing discussions meaningful and valuable. Sometimes there is not enough time to address all the staff items. As the manager, you may need to prioritize requests, but you should communicate your shared concern about the item and ensure staff members it will be on the next agenda.

Staff meetings are an appropriate forum for staff members to share clinical information or "better ways of doing things," or to evaluate any process that affects their patient care or work life. For example, a typical staff meeting may consist of administrative agenda items: addressing the fact that the medical social worker (MSW) is on vacation on such dates and the other MSW who will be covering the clients and available for new referrals, the new home health aide assignment form (the nurses and aides should see drafts first), and any problems that need resolution or clarification.

These meetings can also foster camaraderie and trust among members. Any manager in homecare or hospice knows that the nurses must feel that other staff members are clinical peer professionals, or problems can arise with long-term coverage or assignments. In addition, some nurses have other nurses they usually want to cover their patients if the nurses are sick or on vacation. As long as the

Continued.

THE IMPORTANCE OF STAFF MEETINGS IN HOMECARE AND HOSPICE—cont'd

patient is cared for appropriately and cliques do not develop, nothing is inherently wrong with this practice.

These meetings can also influence positive morale as the nurses in the community realize they are not alone and that the other homecare nurses share the same concerns. Some HHAs hold their meetings at lunchtime and have food there for their staff or the staff brings their own lunch. Others hold meetings in the morning. The common complaint about early morning meetings in homecare is that patients with IVs or receiving insulin must be seen in the morning. Schedule meetings at whatever time seems best for the consensus of the staff. It is difficult, if not impossible, to listen and **hear** what is being said in a staff meeting if the nurse is worried about her next three patients. Always include evening and weekend staff. This allows them a forum for issues even if they are unable to attend.

The manager must value the meetings and thus make them mandatory. Again, it is difficult to hold staff members accountable for what they were not told in the interviewing, hiring, and orientation processes. If a requirement for your program is that staff meetings are mandatory, this needs to be communicated clearly to all. However, the manager must be realistic about such a decision. Obviously, with an extensive traffic back-up or a patient problem in the community needing resolution, the actions of the homecare nurse are clear. However, the nurse should call the manager as soon as possible and explain her absence. Minutes from these meetings should be typed and distributed to staff. This process reinforces items presented and resolves the "I wasn't at the staff meeting" comments and resulting problems.

Again, allow the homecare staff input into the time and, if appropriate, place of the meetings. Try to make these meetings informative and valued. The meetings should start promptly and end at the designated time. If you note many absences, this may be a sign that the staff does not value the time and content of the meetings.

STAFF MEETING EVALUATIONS

Regularly evaluate the staff meetings. On a written evaluation form, ask open-ended questions to elicit if staff needs are being met by the current forum. Some HHAs have only the nurses and home health aides at the meetings, others involve the MSWs as well. These choices and decisions are all based on your program's unique history and needs. Some HHAs do an annual (or more frequently if needed) evaluation of the staff meeting structure, agenda contents, physical space, and so on, to ensure, as part of the CQI process, that meetings are meaningful to all involved.

INTRADISCIPLINARY TEAM CONFERENCES

Some HHAs schedule their intradisciplinary team conferences immediately following the staff meetings. For example, if the staff meeting is held every other Wednesday at 11:30 A.M. and the meeting is conducted during lunch, the clinical case conferences begin promptly at 12:30 P.M., when the other service representatives appear for these meetings. Again, the staff meeting must end promptly, particularly if you are paying to have the professional associates, such as the physical therapist, speech/language pathologist, and the occupational therapist, who are waiting for the nurse and the home health aide who are in the meeting room next door. The rationale for scheduling such conferences in this way is (1) there may be new referrals for these colleagues, and the nurses can expect that they will be able to discuss these new patients with the appropriate colleague after the staff meeting, and (2) the staff members are already out of the field, and to bring them in another day means the nurse is not making needed visits in the community. Always try to get "the most mileage" out of an idea or process. In the above example, the nurses are already at the office. To bring them in another day and disrupt their schedule may not be cost-effective because it pulls the nurse out of the community again.

HOSPICE STAFF SUPPORT

Similarly, some hospices have the ongoing staff support sessions scheduled immediately following their hospice staff meeting. The meeting with the facilitator is scheduled in this way for a few reasons. First, the staff is already on-site, having just attended the staff meeting. Second, the clinical and administrative issues that needed to be addressed were usually taken care of in the staff meeting. The resolution of the problems and the end of the staff meeting helped the staff members let go of those immediate concerns as they were completed. Third, the staff members may be in a more relaxed frame of mind than if they had just driven to the office, ran up the stairs, and sat down for staff support or were late or feel harassed. This also helps ensure that the group is all present at the onset of the meeting, which decreases or minimizes the interruptions or disruptions.

It is important in staff support meetings that the facilitator, the format and process, and the associated environment also be regularly evaluated by the manager and the hospice team participating in hospice support. In homecare and hospice, it is of utmost importance that we care for the caregivers. The stress of the care provided must be identified and dealt with effectively and appropriately. The managers in homecare and hospice must be aware and attuned to the stress levels and any overextension of involvement by the nurse with the patients and their families. For an in-depth review of stress of both manager and staff members, please refer to Chapter 10, "Taking Care of Yourself and Staff."

STAFF MEETINGS WITH ADMINISTRATIVE STAFF MEMBERS

In homecare or hospice you may also have accountability for administration and operations subordinates who report to you. This can include clerical and secretarial staff, scheduling and intake staff, and billing and accounting personnel. Others may include patient coordinators, private pay schedulers, and miscellaneous staff members. It is important to hold meetings with this staff. Initially, meetings should be held weekly, until you understand the paper flow and work process across the organization. It is important that the staff who represent the agency or program on the phone (as well as in person) be articulate, helpful, and professional. Some HHAs have CQI standards for all these functions. An example would be a policy of all phones being answered by the third ring. Referral sources want to call these types of service-driven organizations. Remember, how you sound on the phone forms an outsider's first impression of you. Clearly, a case manager who wants effective care, usually at the "best" price, will call a service-oriented organization. The perception here is that how things "look" is how they are.

All parts of your team must work together. Do not make references to outside (field, visiting) staff and inside (administrative) staffs. The team works together. All team members should be equally busy. In addition, the office administrative staff reporting to you should be cross-trained whenever possible. Always keep this in mind when bringing in new administrative staff members. For example, the clerical staff should be able to enter data on patients as a back up to the billing staff. Remember, many vacations and holidays must be covered. Do not put yourself in the position of having only one person who can do a given function (e.g., data entry, intake, statistical report collation, phones, reception, aide scheduling, record review).

Have your administrative staff function as small teams broken down into similar functions. Cross-train them all to know at least one other position. Do not wait until a crisis to discover the effectiveness of a staff member's cross-training. Plan for practice days and stagger the days so there is backup. These efforts will pay off significantly. It is also a way to develop your staff and see and value them for their range of skills.

Remember, part of your job as manager (and in homecare this is a large part) is to help make the clinical staff members' jobs easier by the successful resolution of administrative problems. For example, if your homecare nurses are being hassled by an archaic or duplicative documentation or operational system, address this concern. Have the administrative and clinical staffs work together with you to determine a more successful way to handle the process.

FISCAL RESPONSIBILITIES IN HOMECARE

In no other setting in health care are the billing functions as closely integrated with the clinical information as in the HHA. Because the HHA must have the physicians's plan of care (POC) on the clinical record before billing for the care provided, this discussion begins with documentation.

Though not all patients are Medicare patients, Medicare sets the standard for documentation, and sometimes coverage, offered by other payors. Because documentation in homecare can comprise an entire book, the following discussion is an overview of the topic to assist the homecare manager develop the staff's documentation skills.

AN OVERVIEW OF HEALTH CARE FINANCING ADMINISTRATION

The Health Care Financing Administration (HCFA) has responsibility for the Medicare and Medicaid programs. Remember that Medicare is a medical insurance program and, like all medical insurers, there are exclusions to coverage of services. HCFA is administratively under the Secretary of Health and Human Services. HCFA contracts with insurance companies to process and adjudicate (make a payment determination or decision) Medicare claims. There are nine Regional Home Health Intermediaries (RHHIs); these process all the home health agency and hospice claims nationally. These RHHIs are generally given the HHAs in certain geographic areas as their service area. (However, chain HHAs usually have one RHHI because these HHAs may have centralized billing).

The HCFA created, with input from HHAs, the current 485/6/7 forms. In addition, the Conditions of Participation (COPs) are also part of Medicare requirements for HHAs. With this information in mind, be aware that HCFA, by law, can pay only for necessary and covered care. When admitting patients to your program, ensure that they meet all the criteria. For example, they must meet the homebound or otherwise meet the skilled care criteria. This criteria must be reflected in the clinical documentation.

DOCUMENTATION

All efficient HHAs must have their nurses and other care providers generate documentation that simultaneously does the following:

1. Demonstrates in the documentation the patient care provided and the patient's response to that care.
2. Shows that current standards of care are maintained.
3. Meets documentation requirements for Medicare and other payors.

The nurse's entries in the patient's clinical record are recognized as a significant contribution that documents the standards of care provided to a patient. As the practice of nursing has become more complex, so, too, have the factors that influence the roles of documentation. Some of these factors include requirements of regulatory agencies (e.g., the State Health Department), health insurance payors (e.g., Medicare), accreditation organizations (e.g., JCAHO, NLN), and consumers of health care and legal entities.

In homecare, the nurse must try to satisfy these various requirements all at once, often with precious few moments in which to accomplish this important task. The book *Handbook of Home Health Standards and Documentation Guidelines for Reimbursement*[2] was written expressly to show how to ensure meeting the various requirements simultaneously. The manager should have these standards and guidelines available to the homecare and discharge planning staff members. This will help ensure an understanding of the level and clarity of specific documentation required by any payor.

As manager, review a percentage of your staff's documentation on an ongoing basis to monitor the quality of care as demonstrated in the documentation and to ensure that other, particularly reimbursement, requirements are being met. This review can also be incorporated into your CQI program, and clinical factors may be identified through the review process that can become the subject of focused studies. In addition, areas for further education may be identified through this process.

In your sample review, ask the questions below to assess the quality of the home care medical record.

NURSE MANAGER'S CHECKLIST FOR DOCUMENTATION

✔ Try to look at the documentation objectively; does it tell the story of the patient's progress (or lack of progress) and the interventions implemented based on the initial assessment and plan of care?

✔ Are telephone calls and other communications with physicians and other team members documented? Do they explain what occurred with the patient, what actions were ordered, modified, and implemented, and the patient's response to these interventions?

✔ Is the nursing process demonstrated in the record? Look for the nursing diagnoses, the assessment, evidence of care planning, implementation of ordered interventions and actions, assessment of the patient's response, and continued evaluation.

✔ Is there documentation of goal achievement and/or progress towards predetermined, mutually set goals and outcomes? Are the goals realistic, quantifiable, and patient-centered?

✔ If progress has not occurred as planned, are the reasons explained in the documentation?

✔ Is the patient's/caregiver response to care interventions or actions documented?

✔ Are the interventions modified, based on the patient's response, where appropriate?

✔ Is there evidence of intradisciplinary team conferences and discussions?

✔ Does the chart show continuity of care planning goals and consistent movement toward goal achievement?

✔ Generally, does the record tell the story of the patient's care and progress while receiving homecare services?

✔ Do the entries and overall information reflect care of the level expected by today's health care consumers and their families?

✔ Finally, does the clinical documentation demonstrate compliance with regulatory, licensure, and quality standards?

16 TIPS TO HELP YOU HELP YOUR STAFF IMPROVE DOCUMENTATION

✔ As a manager, show by your actions that you value effective documentation. This attitude will be conveyed to staff and become the standard of the performance expected.

✔ Remember that writing effective documentation is a learned skill, and, as with any skill, improvement comes only with practice.

✔ Recognize that in homecare, at the first visit the nurse usually begins the process of claims payment (or denial) with the initial 485 and then 486/7 forms.

✔ Have your nurses read their own documentation objectively. They should ask themselves, does this 485/6/7 or visit record say why the patient is homebound (if Medicare or another insurer that has that criteria) and how or why the skills of a nurse or therapist are needed? Involve your staff in peer review of clinical charts. This will significantly help develop their documentation skills, and they will be able to objectively read their own documentation.

✔ As a manager, look at who is admitted to the homecare program. Do the patients meet your admission criteria? (This is also a quality assurance function.) If the nurse cannot clearly identify the skilled, covered service needed but does know the requirements, the patient may not be appropriate for insurance coverage. This patient may still have care needs that another program may provide.

✔ Have your staff focus on the patient's problems in their documentation. That is why homecare is being provided, and it is what the payors must see to justify reimbursement.

✔ Have your nurses demonstrate through their documentation that the care provided is patient-centered. Make the patient goals quantifiable and outcomes patient-centered and specific to the patient's unique problems and needs. Whenever possible, the patient should help set these goals.

✔ Emphasize to the nurses that anyone else who picks up their patient's chart does not have the information they have from actually being there and seeing the patient in their own home setting. Encourage your staff to write information that is objective and clearly paints a picture of the patient, the problems, the needs, and where the care is directed for goal achievement and discharge.

✔ Have the clinical records reviewed overall by the nurse when the initial admitting information has been completed. Use a checklist form to make it easier. This is the best time to check that all identifying information is completed and consistent across the various admission forms. For example, if allergies are noted on the referral information, this same information, after being validated by the patient on the admission visit, should be noted on the medication list and the 485 form (POC). This way, you as the manager know that if the state or HCFA should make an unannounced onsite visit, your charts have met minimal requirements.

✔ Remember to tell your staff that effective documentation does not have to be lengthy or wordy. However, it should convey to any reader the status of your patient, the plan for care, and the consistent movement towards predetermined patient-centered goals.

✔ Have the nurses check that the information on the record flows well and that you can tell by objective evidence what is happening with the patient. This includes the problems, projected plans, and the skilled services that are needed, based on the clear picture presented in the documentation.

✔ Emphasize that paperwork needs to be legible, neat, and organized consistently.

✔ Remind your staff that the payors generally only know as much as is communicated on the 485/6/7 forms. They are painting a picture for the payor/reviewer of why the patient needs nursing or other skilled services. Emphasize that the forms must document why the care was initiated, what the professional nurse is doing (i.e., what are the skilled nursing interventions), where the patient's plan is going (patient-centered goals), and the plans for discharge (rehabilitation potential) and why the case should continue for recertification.

✔ Encourage and appoint a staff nurse representative to your HHA's regularly scheduled CQI committee meetings. This nurse can communicate to peers the important role of documentation.

✔ Instruct your homecare nurses to complete admissions and most of the documentation in the patient's home whenever possible. This is particularly true for new admissions to homecare or hospice care. Patients clearly know that third-party payors (except in private pay service homecare) generally pay for the care the HHA is providing. Complete the 485 and begin the 486 through to item 12 (which is identifying types of information). Complete the visit record and all the initial admitting forms. The nurse should not rely on memory to complete needed documentation. In addition, tell your nurses to explain on the initial visit that requirements must be met for the payors and that the last few minutes of the visit are for the nurse to complete these requirements. Some agencies have implemented this standard very successfully, and it is reflected in the quality of the detailed documentation.

✔ Emphasize that the POC is the most important part of the homecare clinical record. All other information flows from the identified skilled needs ordered on the plan. Hold training sessions on the correct completion of the 485 (and the 486/7). If you identify gaps on the data elements on the POC or if the content is not appropriate or detailed enough for effective patient care, such training will be timely.

THE IMPORTANCE OF REPORTS

Reports present information that is useful and objective for any manager. They track what is happening with the HHA or program.

Many types of report tools are available. Following is a discussion of the report tools the new manager should find helpful. A prudent manager is up to date on the status or health of the HHA. Keeping current helps ensure the early and easy identification of problems or trends that should be watched closely before they become risk management problems or financial disasters. Reports ensure objective findings of different components of the operations in a HHA. This helps the manager by showing information in an organized format that assists and improves managerial effectiveness. Reports can quantify information you may need. For example, if you believe that the nursing visits are up significantly over the last 2 weeks (e.g., by viewing the nurse visit logs or the number of referrals), the actual report that integrates the information by nurse, by week, and by total visits by day or week would validate that finding. This report and the rationale would then help justify an increase in FTEs to your supervisor. The ability to show the increase in care and visits to meet the patient's needs is a key to successful HHA operations.

Management Report Tools for New Managers

1. Use your referral logs as an important source of information at least weekly. The weekly information may be tabulated by your staff for monthly or cumulative reports. Look at:
   - Who and where your referrals are coming from. Are there trends in the diagnoses, types of patients, payor sources, or other information (i.e., visits per referral may indicate level of acuity)?
   - Who are the specific hospitals, physicians, discharge planners, and inpatient nurses? Compare this current information to that of the previous period. If a change exists, try to determine its cause. Have your own HHA coordinator involved in the causes.
   - The referral log's information cannot be underestimated. Use this as a working management tool to track your referrals or nurse care manager caseloads or to project future work assignments. In addition, it is the one place, at a glance, to see your payor mix or geographic spread or to identify trends.
2. Readmission (if within 31 days) to hospital reports.
3. Patient or family complaint logs.
4. Accident/incident logs.
5. HCFA form 488 requests. This is the form generated by the RHHI that requests more clinical information. It should include the date received and the date the information is requested. In addition, look at the entire process: locating, copying, and collating the information. Analyze these findings on a quarterly basis, as these re-

quests for information cost time and money. In addition, share the request with the primary nurse, not in a negative or punitive way, but as an educational opportunity and as a way to perhaps avoid such information requests in the future.

Clearly, an increase in 488 forms may signify the need for in-service training on documentation and the correct completion of the HCFA 485/6/7 forms.

6. Reports generated from automated systems. Many HHAs now have specialized software systems to assist them in their daily operations in such important and time-consuming areas as intake/referrals or billing data entry. Many of these systems are capable of generating useful information for managers. An example is categorizing patients by diagnosis, geographic area, or primary nurse. In addition, nurse productivity reports or financial reports (e.g., status and aging of accounts) assist the manager in planning daily and future operations. Still others include status of budgeted versus actual expenditures and numerous fiscal information. Such reports can be generated for your weekly or monthly review to assist in making decisions.

7. Monthly or quarterly quality report/update/activities. This report should include all continuing education sessions held since the last report and all ongoing research or special-focus studies. These findings, or a synopsis of the findings, may be appropriate for inclusion in the utilization review committee meeting report or in the HHA annual report.

8. Referral source, patient and family satisfaction surveys.

The importance of the information to be found in reports cannot be understated. An effective automated system that meets your HHA's needs can prove invaluable once you and the staff have learned to use it. The following is a brief discussion about these programs and their applicability in homecare.

Automation

The list below is of factors that need to be addressed before purchasing HHA computer software or choosing software vendors. The more defined your needs, requirements, and knowledge on this issue, the better your decision will meet your agency's requirements.

- Volume
- Current paper processes and workflow
- Budget for this endeavor

- Specifically defined primary need(s) for automation (usually began as a needs/wish list)
- The staff component of using the product (e.g., current and new staff computer comfort levels)

Before making any such capital purchase decisions, consider the following. Believing that automation will streamline all operational functions is naive. Undoubtedly, a software system that simultaneously generates the 485/6/7 forms and the Medicare Part A billing form (UB-82/92) is a great idea and clearly cuts down on duplicative paper and errors. But effective automated paper processes must be in place before smooth transition to any new system is possible. There is a wide variance in the products, price, and features of computer systems. The recommendation that you network with other HHA managers is especially true in this area.

Automation in scheduling and particularly in billing is emphasized as HCFA and other payors move toward an electronic, paperless claims process in the effort to cut costs. This has become an especially heightened issue as the U.S. Congress passes legislation to pay electronic media claims (EMC) faster than claims on paper. EMC can include tape-to-tape, on-line, modem, or other electronic routes. The RHHIs are also working toward the goal of increasing EMC claims from HHA and hospice providers.

In addition, as nursing informatics addresses more issues that affect the provision of care in the community and how such automated nursing needs are different, we may see the proliferation of more options to assist professional nurses in their care of patients at home.

SPECIAL PROGRAMS
Hospice

Hospice care is a very special type of care and is now receiving deserved recognition. The nurses, social workers, chaplain, volunteers, and other hospice team members all bring skills to assist patients and their families in meeting their unique needs. This discussion focuses on the special needs unique to hospice management.

Managers in hospice are unique for several reasons, as follow:

1. They provide direction and support to a staff whose patient population, by definition, has an illness of a terminal nature.
2. They interface daily with the processes of dying and death. Therefore the feedback about feelings of anger, denial, and sadness are incorporated into their management role.

3. They must have specialized skills to work successfully with volunteers.
4. They must have training skills to train and successfully maintain volunteers.
5. They must have specialized knowledge of hospice reimbursement systems (e.g., the Medicare Hospice program and all its specific nuances).
6. All these functions demand effective interpersonal communication skills and the ability to talk and teach about hospice factually and sensitively.

In addition, because of the nature of hospice care, funding has historically been problematic. Many hospices are involved in fund raising to support their continued services in communities. The manager in hospice must have or develop the skills to work with fund-raising committee representatives or other associated entities that do this important work for the hospice. There is an ongoing need to be able to articulate clearly the special needs and costs of hospice care.

Hospices must have systems capable of tracking needed information for such important components of hospice care as bereavement counseling and the associated anniversary or remembrance information. In addition, many hospices keep detailed statistics about their programs and the patients and families served in the community. These needs also generate the need for effective tracking through automated systems.

Personal Emergency Response System Programs

Some HHAs also have another special program that is a part of their organization and that the HHA manager may also have responsibility for—the personal emergency response program (PERS).

Such PERS systems are a unique application of technology that allow some patients the ability to remain in their home alone or give them a heightened sense of security. Most nurses in homecare are familiar with this technology, as most have the subscriber (patient) wear the PERS button around the neck or on a belt clip. This technology is tied into the phone system and, once activated, contacts one or more preselected family members or friends of the subscriber to come over immediately. The responders then go to the home, as they have access, and address the problem. Sometimes the responders are municipal services—the fire department or ambulance service. Falls engender the most calls for help in this patient population.

members to ensure patient safety and service with a PERS system. In addition, many of these programs have volunteers who do some of the actual installation and explanation of this important service and technology. Reports should be available to you, as the manager, about the number of subscriber calls, equipment inventory, current or projected purchase needs, public relations associated with the service, and other factors that ensure a safe and responsive program for subscribers and their families and friends.

In addition, most PERS programs have (at least) quarterly meetings that are advisory in nature. They may include the manager, the operators who receive the calls (the response center), a representative of the company that sells and services your PERS equipment, a representative consumer of the service (if possible), the volunteers who assist with the program, and others in the program who are key factors in the effective functioning of this 24-hour service. Some programs have hundreds of these PERS units in the community because the programs allow some frail or elderly people to remain at home. Otherwise, they could not be at home and alone.

The HHA manager may have responsibility for numerous other programs (e.g., Meals on Wheels, private duty services, or durable medical equipment and supply services) in day-to-day operations. With the increasing population of the older elderly (over 85 years), and as community service becomes more the pattern of care, these types of programs can be expected to grow.

A WORD ABOUT HUMAN RESOURCE RECORDS

HHAs maintain files on their personnel. Such files must be maintained in an orderly and consistent method. There should be a standard format for keeping performance evaluations, PPD or x-ray results, status on hepatitis B information, physical, completed safety inservice programs, orientation checklist, and competency evaluations on all employees. This not only reflects internal organization and the value placed on needed detail, but should surveyors or other external visitors appear, you know that all information is complete and in order. A tickler file system can be used to generate a monthly list of information due, including performance evaluations, CPR recertifications, license renewals, PPDs, and so on.

In addition, as part of the CQI program, pull the personnel records of the caregivers noted in the patient clinical records you are reviewing. This is how the surveyor will do it, so practice these methods to identify your internal problems so they are not a bigger problem for the HHA.

Review Chapter 3, Human Resource Management, as it is germane to this discussion about homecare and the special needs of the managers.

SUMMARY

The homecare manager of the future must be flexible, have vision, and be committed to a service-oriented management style. This manager will use newer technologies with the staff to ensure increased communications and safety for the staff. Even 5 years ago, who would have imagined the number of car phones, voice mail, and beepers in use as there are today for homecare staff?

All of those involved with homecare are aware of the incredible growth in dollars, patients, and provided services over the past few years. Homecare and hospice will continue to grow as patients become more proactive consumers—they will continue to demand care in their own home setting. However, as managed care continues to grow and sometimes appears to rachet down the number of patient visits, the homecare manager must be able to articulate the clinical needs of the patient for that patient to receive quality care while remaining at home. Who would have thought that Dobutamine drips, PICC lines, or ventilators would be daily occurrences in homecare? These and other types of complex patient problems will increase as the health care technology explosion continues.

The proactive manager who can quantify and communicate staff needs and explain to superiors the needs based on objective information will be successful in homecare. This chapter is a brief overview of what you need to know to manage a quality program. Many good resources are available to the new manager in homecare. The hope is that you will locate or create them.

REFERENCES

1. Health Insurance Manual—11: Washington, DC, 1989, Government Printing Office.
2. Marrelli TM: Handbook of home health standards and documentation guidelines for reimbursement, St. Louis, 1991, Mosby.

CHAPTER 13

Where To From Here?

T. M. Marrelli

During the course of your career, there may be times when you question your level of job satisfaction. Your questioning might begin in the form of occasional nagging doubts such as, "Why did I ever accept this position?" or "Management is nothing like the recruiter told me it would be." Maybe you find yourself not laughing as much, or dwelling on work problems when at home, or answering the phone at home with the name of your unit. All these are clues that it may be time to reevaluate your job satisfaction. If, like many workers today, you are seeking personal fulfillment, this introspective evaluation may be a difficult process. However, you should start the process when you want to, not when you are stressed out and are forced to address the issue. So where do you start?

Nurses, by nature and education, have a strong tendency to take care of others. However, this chapter's focus is on you and your needs and goals. You must realize that the perfect job does not exist. All positions have their own unique strengths and drawbacks. This review includes what your aspirations were when you accepted your current position, your dreams of being a nurse when you were a student, and your perspectives on the realities of nursing now. Put simply, are your professional and self-fulfillment needs being met in your current position and environment? Are your expectations realistic?

ASSESSING JOB SATISFACTION

The types of questions to ask to assess your satisfaction with your job may be broken down into two areas: (1) the work and the associated environment or culture of the setting in which you manage, and (2) your professional and personal needs and where these fit in your life in relation to other responsibilities. These questions are best answered initially with a quick "yes" or "no" without much thought (this is your "gut" feeling). You can then go back and reconsider your answers after the overall evaluation is complete.

The following questions may help you assess your position and determine if management and this particular position are suitable for you.

THE WORK AND ITS ENVIRONMENT

✔ Do you enjoy the actual work tasks? In management this includes the human management activities of dealing with difficult personalities, conflict resolution, and having the position of power (whether or not you want it). This also includes the satisfaction of being part of a special team providing care to patients and being able to effect needed change or being appreciated by patients' families.

✔ Overall, do you like going to your job every day?

✔ Do you feel you have some control over outcomes and the tasks accomplished?

✔ Generally, are the obstacles to completion outweighed by the work accomplished?

✔ Generally, do you feel that you have the support you need to accomplish your work? If you decide that you enjoy the actual work responsibilities but still are not happy at work, consider whether your supervisor provides sufficient support for your team to get tasks accomplished. Continual frustration of goal achievement is very disheartening and leads to nurse manager and staff turnover. You may wonder, "Who else cares, so why should I?"

✔ Does your job leave you feeling energized or drained? Does your family see you enough? When they do, are you emotionally available, or are you redoing the staffing schedule in your head while having dinner?

It is important to note that some of us have a tendency to give and take care of everyone and everything except ourselves. This can lead to exhaustion and burnout if we do not take steps to care for ourselves. Our work life must be successfully integrated into other parts of our lives.

Part of the personal growth process is the identification of problem areas in our lives and the identification of actions for resolution. Maslow's needs identify the basic needs that must initially be attained before self- actualization can be achieved. The setting, evaluation, and reevaluation of personal and professional goals on a regular basis can be an effective tool in achieving what we want.

YOUR PERSONAL NEEDS

✔ Do you find the actual activities of the manager stimulating while being able to integrate the rest of your responsibilities into your life (such as your family and friends)?

✔ Are the rewards appropriate to the energy expended?

✔ Are you able to fulfill your own personal goals in this position (e.g., go back to school, have a family, complete certification, teach Sunday school class, or be a volunteer firefighter or paramedic in your community)?

Focus on the answers to these questions. The direction your career takes is up to you. It is always okay to reconsider and ultimately readjust career goals to meet your unique needs. After a thorough review of your answers, your next step is to reaffirm or reevaluate your stated goals. In this way you can begin implementing changes to work toward achieving them. Only you know what will contribute to the feeling of self-fillment in your life. It has been said that, "Nurses leave the profession because they experience a lack of personal fulfillment, stemming from their inability to meet the unrealistic expectations imposed by this ever-changing environment."[1] Nurse managers do not always have to leave their current work environment to feel more fulfilled in their professional roles. Skills that nurses use daily outside the work realm lend themselves to other potentially fulfilling professional or personal activities. The following are examples of such endeavors:

1. *Organizational skills*—Are you the family member who is, by nature, the organizer? You can use these skills in professional association activities in various administrative capacities.
2. *Writing skills*—Do you edit the community newsletter or contribute to the local newspaper? This can be developed into a resource for the nursing news at your facility or for publication in a professional nursing journal.
3. *Public speaking skills*—This needed communication skill can be used by speaker's bureaus, the local community college for health classes, support groups, or for speeches to elementary school students on subjects such as, "Why I Like Being a Nurse."
4. *Persuasive skills*—Consider running for office or campaigning for the candidate of your choice.

Any of these special skills can be effective in assisting you in meeting your goals and helping you match them with your unique talents.

In the beginning of this chapter, you evaluated your satisfaction with your current work position and where it fits in your life. This chapter also discusses the importance of recognizing available employment choices. Specific ways to succeed and make yourself uniquely qualified for a position are addressed, and examples of choices and qualifications that may be helpful to you are included.

CHOICES

Choices are options that you give yourself. People tend not to give themselves the luxury of choices. In addition, even when we know that we may be unhappy in our work environment, we may procrastinate about taking the steps needed to change and grow. You are not alone. (The Procrastinator's Club has approximately 10,000 members!)

Once you recognize that professional nurses have numerous choices for employment, you can begin to explore your many options. Even if you have a satisfying job, considering your options can provide growth opportunities important to your professional career in the future. This is also a way to help market yourself and your skills. Being open to and considering your choices enables you to (1) keep some perspective on your current job (this is particularly important when you are unhappy in your position), (2) receive objective feedback about yourself and the external professional environment, and (3) receive information on possibilities for the future. This feedback can be received through the interview process, through networking with professional associates, and through other methods of communication.

MARKETING YOURSELF

Marketing is broadly defined as the theory and practice of selling. In reality, we market ourselves in any interpersonal or written encounter. However, when we consciously market ourselves, we focus on the unique skills that we bring to a work environment and offer to a prospective employer, enhancing our desirability to that employer. Examples of assets that make a nurse uniquely qualified include advanced degrees or certification in a specialty area. Still other examples include awards, experience, and other types of recognition in a chosen field. We sometimes tend to underestimate our own unique skills. The credit and acknowledgment of others can be of important benefit in achieving your long-term professional goals.

A large part of successfully marketing yourself is your projection of your belief in yourself. This is your self-confidence. We know that feelings follow thoughts. Therefore, even if on a bad day you are not feeling self-assured, your acting that way may contribute to your feeling more confident. Use available resources to develop or improve such self-promoting skills. Look at role models who seem self-assured; watch how they act, dress, and behave. It is important that you recognize your strengths and areas for improvement. This level of self-knowledge leads to an increased self-assurance that is communicated as belief in yourself.

IDENTIFYING YOUR UNIQUE OR SPECIAL SKILLS

Though professional RNs must pass nursing boards for licensure, and thus meet specific standards, the following section addresses additional ways to help you grow professionally.

Certification

In the 1940s, nurse anesthetists were the first nurses required to meet specific standards to enter professional practice. Since then, certification has grown to encompass those nurses who meet high standards through experience and expertise in nursing practice. Certification is a validation of clinical or administrative skill. The process of certification generally requires an RN license, a set amount of years or hours in practice in a specific specialty, and documented continuing education credit hours. A major benefit of professional certification is the recognition that sets certified nurses apart. Several nursing organizations have boards for certifying nurses. These boards set the criteria, determine scoring, validate credentials, and confer certification in over 50 nursing specialties. Examples of organizations that certify nurses include the ANA, the American Association of Critical Care Nurses, and the National Certification Corporation. These and other unique credentials you have as a nurse contribute to your power base as a nurse and nurse manager. Refer to the section on Resources for Further Professional Development at the end of the book for more information.

Writing for Professional Publication

Because of their clinical expertise and communication skills, all nurses, particularly those in management, have something important to share with other nurses and nurse managers. In addition, the initiative and perseverance necessary to research and develop an idea and then create and submit a completed manuscript reflect other desirable traits to a prospective employer. Publication in a nursing journal, for example, sets you apart from other candidates who may be similarly qualified. This has been particularly true for some time in the academic environment.

Workshops, Seminars, and Other Development Activities

Some people attend classes and expect to absorb all the information by listening quietly. Yet, it has been demonstrated that we forget most of what we learn within days, particularly when there is no active participation on our part. The following 10 tips can help you make the most of learning and networking opportunities at professional workshops or seminars.

10 TIPS FOR LEARNING

✔ Set three learning goals. Develop a list of three to six overall goals in attending the educational session. This will help you focus your thinking. Your goals generally will be oriented toward getting specific questions answered or utilization or practical application of skills or theory.

✔ Think about specific questions you want answered. Develop a list of 10 to 15 specific questions. (Consider giving this list to the seminar leader(s) in advance.)

✔ Meet other participants at the program. Talk to them. Each attendee has a specific area of expertise. Make a note of it. Start your own network. Exchange cards (bring along plenty). Go to breakfast, lunch, and dinner with those with whom you can share information and learn.

✔ Develop a plan of action. Make a list of anything you want to consider doing differently when you get back on the job. This will help you apply what you learned and help you achieve objective benefits.

✔ Participate. Ask questions and make contributions. Comment. Be visible. You will benefit in two ways. First, your mind will almost automatically start working on information, problems, and solutions. Second, the speaker and other attendees will also contribute by finding answers for you.

✔ Make contact with the seminar leader personally (and early) when possible. She or he will think more of and about you. It will also be easier to follow up with questions and problems after the program.

✔ Take clear, detailed notes. Not only will this be helpful for future reference, but the very act of taking good notes and organizing your thoughts will keep you more involved. Take notes legibly and coherently the first time to eliminate any need for rewriting them later.

✔ Write a brief report—one to three pages—based on your plan of action and notes. Consider sharing your report with your supervisor.

✔ Hold a staff meeting when you get back and share the useful information you have gained. Implement a plan of action using your new ideas.

✔ Enjoy yourself—we all learn more when we are having a good time.

NETWORKING

The contacts made and developed through professional organizations can be very advantageous. In time, these professional colleagues may become your peer support group, your friends, and sources of information on viable job alternatives when you want to move on professionally.

RESUMES AND CURRICULUM VITAE

Resumes, curriculum vitae, and associated cover letters all represent you. Remember, they are sometimes the only communication about you that a prospective employer receives. These first impressions do count. Resumes are used in most business settings, whereas curriculum vitae are used primarily in the educational and teaching realms. Always type your resume or curriculum vitae, and print the document on the best quality paper available. It is a good idea to have someone proofread your resume or curriculum vitae and cover letter for content, implications, format, clarity, and typographic errors. If no one is available to provide objective comments, put your materials aside for a day or two and then reread them. You may be amazed at the findings. Most print or copy shops will print your resume or curriculum vitae on quality paper fairly inexpensively. The outcome may be worth the cost if it results in additional interviews scheduled. About now, you might be saying, "I do not have the time to do all this and pay attention to such details." Remember the resumes and cover letters that have come across your desk? You have probably been drawn to those that are short and neat, and that communicate clearly. Use your time management skills to ensure that the documents you provide any perspective employer are clear, complete, accurate, and professional.

Your resume, particularly for management positions, should indicate the number and types of staffs you have been responsible for in your current and previous positions. Be clear about your level of responsibility—e.g., "24-hour responsibility for over 50 nurses and for over 25 professional associates (speech-language pathologists, occupational therapists, medical social workers, physical therapists, etc.) who cared for over 400 patients in the home setting." When writing your resume, always use verbs that express management in action. Appropriate verbs are *created, developed, implemented, evaluated, supervised, problem solved, analyzed,* etc. Many good books on resume writing are available, and a few are listed in the resources section at the end of the book. An example of a cover letter, the introductory

---

EXAMPLE OF A COVER LETTER

June 14, 199●

Alice Campbell, RN, MSN
Recruitment Office
St. Elsewhere General Hospital
Anytown, Maryland 11111-2222

1212 Mockingbird Lane
Anytown, Maryland 11111-2222

Dear Ms. Campbell,

I am writing in response to your ad for a nurse manager in the Sunday Anywhere Paper of June 12, 1994. I believe my 4 years of experience in the St. Elsewhere General Hospital telemetry unit as evening shift coordinator, as well as other accomplishments, make me uniquely qualified for this position.

I have attached my resume, which highlights my experience, for your confidential review. I look forward to hearing from you. I can be reached at (410) 222-1234.

Sincerely,

Jennifer Brown, RN

---

letter about you and your skills that accompanies your resume or curriculum vitae, is given in the box.

BEFORE THE INTERVIEW

Consider *any* communication that occurs with a prospective employer as an opportunity to shine and market yourself. Even if you suspect that the employer may not be considering you or have a position available for someone with your unique qualifications, remember that this person might consider you in the future. What you do and say today can position you for a future job. Your interactions can influence early deliberations about such future opportunities.

At the beginning of this chapter you considered and identified what is important in order for you to meet your unique needs in a nursing position. The following sections will discuss the active process of the job search and offer tips for finding and getting the job you want.

PREPARING FOR THE INTERVIEW

✔ Find out all you can about your prospective employer.

✔ Talk to employees, including nurses you know who no longer work there.

✔ Recognize that the advertisements in the newspaper communicate important information about the position and the facility. For example, does the ad describe where you would live and work geographically (urban, rural, etc.)? Does the employer sound progressive? Does the ad mention clinical ladders, collaborative practice models, or other progressive nurse-oriented activities that are important to you? Ads sometimes communicate the management philosophy. Ads may provide information that can help you determine whether or not you would fit in as a team member in a particular setting.

✔ Obtain written materials. Most health care facilities produce flyers or brochures, available to the community, about their services. Read the factual information listed. This may include the size of the facility or program, the number of beds (if an in-patient setting), the mission statement or goals, the specific services or programs provided (e.g., maternity care, ambulatory care, hospice, home health), and the geographic area they serve.

✔ Write and send a cover letter with your resume to the person identified in the newspaper ad. This may be the nurse recruiter, the nursing office supervisor, or an administrator for the clinical area. In the letter clearly request consideration and an interview at this person's earliest convenience. Set the tone to sound professional and enthusiastic.

✔ Think about and prepare a written list of questions for the interview. Your questions might relate to the nursing philosophy, the mission statement of the program, the average staffing ratios on the unit you would be managing, the kind of documentation system used, computerization status, the average length of stay for the hospital or for the specific unit, or information about the nursing newsletter.

✔ Make a list of questions you think you might be asked and practice answering them. Think of those questions that you ask prospective applicants. Practice before the interview so that you will not need to have your notes with you. Questions commonly asked in interviews include:

- ✔ Where do you want to be professionally in 5 or 10 years?
- ✔ What are your strengths and weaknesses?
- ✔ Give an example of a particularly difficult management situation and how you addressed the problem.
- ✔ Why are you looking for another position?
- ✔ Tell me about your nursing management style.
- ✔ Why do you want to work here?
- ✔ What is your background ?
- ✔ Why do you believe you are the best person for this job?

Your responses should reflect your professionalism, job knowledge, management skills, and goals. Being well prepared will also help decrease any interview jitters or nervousness.

THE INTERVIEW

The interview process is appropriately valued as the most important factor in getting a job. In addition, the interview is an important step in the information-gathering process about the prospective employer. Through active listening to someone who knows the system and manages there, you can learn needed information about the actual nursing and management philosophy.

GENERAL TIPS FOR INTERVIEWING

- ✔ The more prepared you are, the more self-assured you will be, and this will be projected to any prospective employer.
- ✔ It is a good idea to bring along an extra resume should the interviewer not be able to locate his or her copy. (If this happens, it may give you important insight into the work environ-

ment, such as disorganization, tight resources, or poor communication between human resources and nursing [or it may be that this is just a bad day].)

✔ It is okay to ask for a copy of the specific position description should one not be offered. Since usually more functions are required than those listed on the position description, consider asking the interviewer to describe the daily routine of the area.

✔ As part of your preparation, bring a typed list of professional and personal references. List the names, professional degrees, addresses, and telephone numbers of your references. The three professional references should be people you have worked with and/or who have supervised your work. Be sure to notify your references that you will be actively interviewing and that they may receive a call. Of course, you should ask if they are willing to serve as references before you list them.

✔ It is important that you appear as calm and composed as you can for an interview. This gets harder the more you want a specific job. Therefore plan to arrive at the setting at least 20 minutes ahead of time, assume you will not find a parking place anywhere near the facility, and plan to complete some paperwork, such as an application, before the actual interview begins.

✔ Be punctual, dress professionally in a suit that you feel good in, get a good night's sleep the night before, and tell yourself that you will have a successful interview.

✔ Use your interpersonal skills and good judgment throughout the process. Allot plenty of time; some interviews can be lengthy depending on who else the interviewer wants you to meet with or on whether the interviewer gives you a tour of the clinical setting.

MAKING THE MOST OF THE INTERVIEW

✔ Use your active listening skills.

✔ If you determine that the interviewer is having a bad day and seems very hassled (e.g., there may be numerous interruptions), know that this could be indicative of the interviewer's personality or of the setting. Try to use your intuitive skills during this encounter to know the difference between a bad day and what is "normal" for the functioning of the setting (e.g., crisis management).

✔ Do not smoke (even if the option is offered).

✔ Try to bring the conversation to the style of management practiced (e.g., "Are the staff nurses involved in shared governance or other aspects of departmental decision making?").

✔ Do not share negative feelings or experiences about your current or past work settings. Although these occur to all of us, discussing them, particularly during a first meeting, may be perceived as indicating failure to appropriately address and handle identified problems.

✔ Act enthusiastic, and you will feel that way. This will be communicated.

✔ Smile, use eye contact appropriately, take some deep breaths, try to relax, and listen.

✔ Communicate to the interviewer that you want this job (if indeed you want it) and that you are right for it.

CONCLUDING THE INTERVIEW

✔ Allow the interviewer to wrap up the interview.

✔ Make sure that your correct phone number is on your resume and application.

✔ Have your questions ready when the interviewer asks, "Do you have any questions for me that I have not covered?"

✔ Thank the interviewer for the time and information.

✔ Ask how soon a decision will be made or what the next step will be (e.g., how soon the interviewer plans to fill the position and when you will be hearing about the decision or a second interview). In addition, ask who you will be hearing from (e.g., the interviewer or the nurse recruiter).

✔ Offer a verbal affirmation of wanting the job at the end of the interview (if you do, or think you do).

THE INTERVIEW WITH YOUR PROSPECTIVE NEW STAFF

Many employers now schedule the nurse manager candidate finalists to meet with and be interviewed by representatives of the staff they may be managing on accepting the position. Usually the staff chooses representatives. The number may vary based on the facility's philosophy. This can be a very useful opportunity for the prospective nurse manager to determine more about the actual day-to-day operations and culture of the clinical area. Usually the nurses chosen are leaders in the staff hierarchy. The interview with representatives of your prospective staff will also give you needed information about the staff and should be looked on as a positive and information-finding meeting. This is your time to be professional, positive, and persuasive. You might practice with a trusted friend the speech about why you are the best candidate for the job and about your style of management.

FOLLOWING UP THE INTERVIEW

If the interviewer or the nurse recruiter does not call by the discussed date, call him or her to determine whether or not a decision has been made and, if not, when you should call back. When you call, be brief and pleasant. Communicate that you are still interested in the position and want to know if a candidate has been selected. Offer to call back the following week. Remember that if you really want the job, be assertive and let the interviewer know that you are available for a second interview if he or she so desires. It is important to be patient. Getting the position you want may take time but will be well worth the wait if the position meets your identified needs.

THANK-YOU LETTERS

Send a thank-you letter to the interviewer within a week after the interview. Even when you call and speak to the interviewer, it is courteous to follow up with a letter. Two sample thank-you letters are provided on p. 303. One gives you an idea of what to say if you are certain you are not interested in the position.

SAMPLE THANK-YOU LETTER

June 21, 199●

Alice Campbell, RN, MSN   1212 Mockingbird Lane
Recruitment Office   Anytown, Maryland 11111-2222
St. Elsewhere General Hospital
Anytown, Maryland 11111-2222

Dear Ms. Campbell:

Thank you for interviewing me yesterday for the position of nurse manager on the B-4 telemetry unit. As you know, I am very interested in assuming this position. I believe I have the skills and experience to be a great asset to St. Elsewhere General Hospital and would welcome the opportunity to join the management team.

I look forward to hearing from you; I can be reached at (410) 222-1234.

Sincerely,

Jennifer Brown, RN

SAMPLE THANK-YOU LETTER

June 21, 199●

Alice Campbell, RN, MSN   1212 Mockingbird Lane
Recruitment Office   Anytown Maryland 11111-2222
St. Elsewhere General Hospital
Anytown, Maryland 11111-2222

Dear Ms. Campbell:

As I said in today's phone conversation, and after further thoughtful consideration, I realize that the nurse manager position is not the job I am seeking at this time. It sounds as if you have a great team working on the B-4 telemetry unit. Thank you for your time. I wish you success in filling your open position and in your other professional endeavors.

Sincerely,

Jennifer Brown, RN

KEEPING A RECORD OF YOUR JOB SEARCH AND INTERVIEW INFORMATION

In your search, you will be in contact with and interviewed by various prospective employers. While you are trying to determine why you prefer one position or setting over another, it can be difficult to remember your thoughts and impressions without a written record. A notebook or log can be an easy way to help you remember details and your overall reactions to a specific facility.

Columns can be drawn vertically down a page with the following kinds of overhead information across the top horizontally. An example is:

Name of facility   Interviewer   Benefits   Follow-up   Outcome

Other variables that may be tracked in the log or notebook include dates (or copies) of letters, positions interviewed for, parking problems, commute time, the actual physical plant, other perceptions, and the interviewer's management or organizational style. Your record could also include your perceptions of such things as the level of cooperation when you called the facility, the human resources office, the security guards, the interviewer's receptionist, and how long you were kept waiting. Overall, did you feel like an intruder or that they were glad to have a promising candidate and communicated that to you? It is hard to go back and recreate details, so keeping the log in the car with you enables you to write your perceptions and objective facts immediately following the interview.

AFTER THE INTERVIEW

Identify whether this position has the critical job elements needed to make you happy and feel as if your best skills are being used. Brainstorm those factors you identified in your self-evaluation process that would help you achieve your professional goals. These may include the location (state, city, rural, urban, etc.), staff development program, professional growth opportunities, and any other factors, such as shared governance or nursing representation at the board level, that you value as criteria preferred in a prospective work setting.

NEGOTIATING

Salary is not the determinant of the best job, but in nursing, as in other fields, it sometimes can be a harbinger of the amount of work you will be responsible for. In addition, although starting nurses' salaries are usually fixed, experienced nurses, particularly managers, may consider negotiating for more based on their unique qualifications. Remember that you may never get what you do not request. Assessing a prospective employer's needs gives you information on which skills to emphasize. Remember:

1. You both want something. You want a fulfilling position that uses your talents effectively, and they want a competent manager who has the skills needed to accomplish the work at hand.
2. You are a competent manager who brings experience to this position. Be positive and enthusiastic about the position, and stress what you can do for them.
3. Know their specific needs. Often in an interview, the interviewer will share information about where the unit or organization is going. In fact, if this information is not shared, this is a good question to ask when the interviewer asks if you have any questions. The actual question could be phrased as, "What is St. Elsewhere General Hospital's vision for the future?" Many times you can use this information to promote your qualifications that make you the best candidate for the position. The following are examples:

HOW ASKING ABOUT THE INSTITUTIONS CAN HELP YOU WIN THE JOB

✔ The interviewer states that the facility is currently completing long-term plans for one of their medical-surgical units to become a designated hospice unit. She or he goes on to say that it looks as if the state planning process is almost completed and that conversion could occur as soon as three months from now. If you have the skills or experience and express the desire to be of assistance, this could place you at an advantage over other candidates. In addition, in this current era of working to increase effectiveness with fewer resources, you could offer this prospective employer flexibility and options they may need.

✔ The interviewer shares the information that they are undergoing a transition to make all the units more decentralized and autonomous. If you have experienced a similar process at another setting, your special knowledge could be valuable to a new employer to help ensure a successful change.

> ✔ Do not be afraid to share your accomplishments. Remember that the resume is only the introduction that gets your foot in the door. There is much more that must be communicated. Identify your special skills and accomplishments, such as serving on the local health department board, being a member of a speaking organization or a speaker's bureau, attaining certification, and publishing. (These special skills and accomplishments should be listed on your resume.)

Before you accept a position, know what you need to be happy and to meet your goals. You may need to negotiate for what you want. People do respect people who negotiate for what they believe they deserve. Many settings now offer "cafeteria style" benefit packages to more successfully meet an individual's needs. This contributes to position retention. Some of these items may be the salary, tuition reimbursement, professional workshops and development, or flexibility in your work hours. Remember that successful negotiations are "win/win"; i.e., you both get what you want.

WHEN YOU RECEIVE AN OFFER

Listen to what is said, and know that you do not have to make a decision immediately. In fact, it may be helpful to "try on" what it would feel like to work at the facility for a few days before giving them an answer. This could include driving the 20 miles to the prospective setting for a few consecutive days to see if the commute would be a problem or other behaviors that might help you in your decision-making process.

ACCEPTING AN OFFER

The job acceptance process can be as individual as the work setting. However, to protect yourself, as a general rule, ask to receive the offer in writing and wait until you receive a written validation of your job offer from your new employer before giving notice to your current employer. This should be done even in instances when the position has been offered verbally and you have verbally accepted. It has happened in some settings that because of disorganization or a miscommunication, it was said that the offer never was extended. If this occurs, it does not matter why it happened; you still do not have the job and will not be working there.

GIVING NOTICE

Read your facility's manual about the procedure for giving notice of resignation in your particular setting. This usually ranges from 2 to 4 weeks depending on the setting and culture. If you have signed a contract, consult your contract. In addition, some nursing agencies, particularly in the sales or community health setting, may have non-compete clauses as part of the nurse's contract or as a separate agreement that was signed on employment. You must address these and other unique situations for your own protection and for professional integrity.

SAMPLE RESIGNATION LETTER

The actual resignation letter can be brief and to the point. Your letter should be directed to your immediate supervisor. The following is an example of the language that should be clearly stated:

"It is with regret that I inform you that effective (specify date), I will be resigning from my position as (position, unit)."

Some people also state that they have enjoyed working in their position, when this is appropriate. It may not be appropriate if your supervisor knows that you have been stressed out and looking for a position for some time.

ABOUT "NOT BURNING BRIDGES"

All managers grow and change and sometimes need to move on, but we have all heard the saying "never burn bridges." This is true in all industries, but particularly in the nursing profession. The cohesiveness of the nursing profession, particularly in one specialty or state, ensures that in the future there will be interaction with past employers. For these reasons, and for your own professional growth, always try to leave the area for which you were responsible in better shape than when you first took the position. This will help you be successful in your future professional endeavors.

GUILT AND GROOMING YOUR SUCCESSOR

Supervisors may try to make you feel guilty once you have made the decision to leave official. You have been in their shoes as a manager, so you already bring insight into this common phenomenon. One way to assuage any guilty feelings you may have is to have already begun the process of developing skills in a few nurses who will be ready to assume your role. When your manager says, "You know I can't fill your position for at least (hyperinflated) weeks and besides . . .," you can offer a suggestion for an appropriate successor. If you have used effective team-building and participatory management skills, your group is sure to have a few staff members qualified to act in your position should there be a delay in replacing you. Remember that you have a choice about whether or not to accept guilt about leaving a job.

SUMMARY

Changes and choices can be difficult but do present new opportunities for growth. Personal and professional development, active involvement in professional nursing associations, and networking with leaders in your specialty field can be occasions for growth. The process of learning, integrating new behaviors, and changing positions can be difficult. Once the choice has been made to accept a new opportunity, you have the challenge of creating a special environment for your team where your management style blends with your employer's organizational goals. Remember that effective nurse managers have been described as a "wonder in action." Being a nurse manager can be very fulfilling and exciting. You may have the good fortune of working with a highly competent and sensitive team.

There is no perfect job, only jobs that meet your needs and aspirations at particular times in your life. Only you can evaluate your unique needs, goals, and dreams and work toward achieving them.

REFERENCES

1. Butler J, Parsons RJ: Hospital perceptions of job satisfaction, *Nurs Manage* 20(8):46, 1989.

2. Patz J, Biordi O, Holm K: Middle nurse manager Effectiveness, *J Nurs Adm* 21(1):15-24, 1991.

Resources for Further Professional Development

Journals and Newsletters

The following journals and newsletters focus on issues and concerns relevant to nurse managers.

JONA (J.B. Lippincott Company, 12107 Insurance Way, Hagerstown, MD 21740, [800] 638-3030)

Nursing Administration Quarterly (Aspen Publishers, Inc., 200 Orchard Ridge Drive, Suite 200, Gaithersburg, MD 20878, [800] 638-8437)

Nursing Economic$ (Anthony J. Jannetti, Inc., North Woodbury Road/Box 56, Pitman, NJ 08071, [609] 589-2319)

Nursing Management (S-N Publications, Inc., 103 North Second Street, Suite 200, Dundee, IL 60118, [708] 426-6100)

Nursing Quality Connection (Mosby–Year Book, Inc., 11830 Westline Industrial Drive, St. Louis, MO 63146, [800] 325-4177)

Conferences

Annual nursing management conferences are sponsored by the following organizations. For further information, please contact the organization.

American Organization of Nurse Executives annual convention (850 North Lake Shore Drive, Chicago, IL 60611, [312] 280-6000)
(State organizations of nurse executives also typically hold conventions and/or conferences.)

Management Conference (annual) (Continuing Nursing Education, Medical College of Pennsylvania, P.O. Box 12608, Philadelphia, PA 19129, [800] 666-7737)

Management Development Annual Conference (Resource Applications/Mosby–Year Book, Inc., 7250 Parkway Drive, Suite 510, Hanover, MD 21076, [800] 826-1877)

Nursing Economic$ annual conference (Anthony J. Jannetti, Inc., North Woodbury Road/Box 56, Pitman, NJ 08071, [609] 589- 2319)

Nursing Management (S-N Publications, Inc., 103 North Second Street, Suite 200, Dundee, IL 60118, [708] 426- 6100)

Certification

The American Nurses Association Credentialing center offers two nursing administration certification programs. They are briefly described below.

Nursing Administration (CNA certification)
The certification offering in Nursing Administration is available to nurses who hold an active RN license in the United States or its territories, who hold a baccalaureate or higher degree, and who hold (or have held) an administrative position at the nurse manager level or the nurse executive level for at least the equivalent of 24 months of full-time service within the past 5 years. The administrative position must be within a health care organization in which clinical nursing services are provided.

Nursing Administration, Advanced (CNAA certification)
The certification offering in Nursing Administration, Advanced, is available to nurses who hold an active RN license in the United States or its territories, who hold a master's or higher degree, and who hold (or have held) an administrative position at the nurse executive level or who have provided consultative services at the nurse executive level for at least the equivalent of 24 months of full-time service within the past 5 years. The administrative position or consultative services must be within a health care organization in which clinical nursing services are provided.

For further information, contact:
American Nurses Association Credentialing Center
1101 14th Street
Washington, DC 20005
(800) 274-4262

Organization Resources: Homecare and Hospice

The following organizations are specific to homecare and hospice and may be helpful for reference:

The National Association for Home Care
519 C St., N.E.
Washington, DC 20002
(202) 547-7424

Foundation for Hospice and Home Care
519 C St., N.E.
Washington, DC 20002
(202) 547-6586
The National Hospice Organization
301 Maple Ave., W, Suite 506
Vienna, VA 22180
(703) 938-4449
American Federation of Home Health Agencies
1320 Fenwick Ln, Suite 100
Silver Spring, MD 20910
(301) 588-1454
Visiting Nurse Associations of America
3801 E. Florida, Suite 900
Denver, CO 80210
(303) 753-0218

FOR FURTHER READING

Chapter 1/The Nurse Manager Role Today

Curtin L: Political savvy, *Nurs Manage* 13(3):7-8, 1982.

Del Bueno DJ: Power and politics in organizations, *Nurs Outlook* 43(3):124-128, 1986.

Gardner KL, Gander M: Transition: from clinician to administrator, *Nurs Manage* 23(1):38-39, 1992.

Hamilton JM, Kiefer ME: Personal power: your key to success, *Nurs 90* pp 146-148, Oct 1990.

Hansten RI: Revisit your sources, *Am J Nurs* 92(1):61- 62, 1992.

Hansten R, Washburn M: Delegation: how to deliver care through others, *Am J Nurs* 92(3):87-90, March 1992.

Harbin R: Practicing effective delegation, *Pediatr Nurs* 16(1):91-92, 1990.

Manthey M: The art of management— three simple rules, *Nurs Manage* 21(1):19-20, 1990.

Manthey M: From "mama management" to team spirit, *Nurs Manage* 21(1):20-21, 1990.

Marriner-Tomey A: *Guide to nursing management*, ed 4, St Louis, 1992, Mosby–Year Book.

Patz JM et al: Middle nurse manager effectiveness, *JONA* 21(1):15-24, 1991.

Peters T, Austin N: *A passion for excellence*, New York, 1985, Random House.

Peters TJ, Waterman RH Jr: *In search of excellence*, New York, 1984, Warner Books.

Veehoff DC: Whole brain thinking and the nurse manager, *Nurs Manage* 23(8):33-34, 1992.

Werkheiser L et al: New nurse managers. I. Orientation for the 1990s, *Nurs Manage* 21(11):56-63, 1990.

Werkheiser L et al: New nurse managers. II. The nurse manager resource peer, *Nurs Manage* 21(12):30-33, 1990.

Chapter 2/Management: An Overview

Blanchard K, Johnson S: *The one minute manager,* New York, 1982, William Morrow.

Blanchard KB, Lorber R: *Putting the one minute manager to work,* New York, 1987, William Morrow.

Darling LW: The mentoring dimension, mentor types and life cycles, Mentoring Series, *JONA* 14(10):43-44, 1984.

Davidhizer R: Managerial credibility, *Nurs Adm Q* 13(3):17-22, 1989.

Douglas L: *The effective nurse: leader and manager,* St Louis, 1984, Mosby–Year Book.

Drucker PF: *Managing for results,* New York, 1984, Harper & Row.

Etzioni A: Humble decision making, *Harvard Bus Rev* 21(2):69-71, 1989.

Gillies DA: *Nursing management—a systems approach,* Philadelphia, 1982, WB Saunders.

Kosowski M et al: An interactive model of leadership, *Nurs Adm Q* 15(1):36-43, 1990.

Kramer M: Trends to watch at the magnet hospital, *Nurs 90* 20(6):67-74, 1990.

Manthey M: The art of management: three simple rules, *Nurs Manage* 21(12):19-20, 1990.

Moloney M: *Leadership in nursing: theory, strategies, action,* St Louis, 1979, Mosby–Year Book.

O'Neil KK, Gajdostik KL: The head nurse's managerial role, *Nurs Manage* 20(6):39-41, 1989.

Orth CD et al: The manager's role as coach and mentor, *JONA* 20(9):11-15, 1990.

Phifer L: Managerial leaders and their influence in nursing, *Pediatr Nurs* 16(3):222, 1990.

Prestholdt C: Modern mentoring: strategies for developing contemporary nursing leadership, *Nurs Adm Q* 15(1).

Rosener JB: Ways women lead, *Harvard Bus Rev,* 68(6):119-125, 1990.

Smith HL, et al: A retrospective on Japanese management in nursing, *JONA* 19(1):27-37, 1989.

Stachura LM, Hoff J: Toward achievement of mentoring for nurses, *Nurs Adm Q* 15(1):56-62, 1990.

Synowiez BB, Synowiez PM: Delphi forecasting as a planning tool, *Nurs Manage* 21(4):18-19, 1990.

Walton M: *The Deming management method,* New York, 1986, Dodd, Mead.

Chapter 3/Human Resource Management

Boyd C et al: Performance plan: a nursing management strategy to improve care delivery, *J Healthcare Educ Train* 5(3):12-15, 1991.

Davidhizar R, Giger J: When subordinates go over your head—the manipulative employee, *JONA* 20(9):29-34, 1990.

Del Bueno DJ, Walker DD: Developing prospective managers: a unique program, part I, *JONA* 14(4):7-10, 1984.

Fulghum R: *All I really need to know I learned in kindergarten,* Westminister, Md, 1988, Villiard Books, Random House.

King P: *Performance planning and appraisal: a how-to book for managers,* New York, 1984, McGraw-Hill.

Lachman VD: Increasing productivity through performance evaluation, *JONA* 14(12):7-14, 1984.

Lawler T: The objectives of performance appraisal or "where can we go from here?" *Nurs Manage* 19(3):82-88, 1988.

Livingston JS: Pygmalion in management, *Harvard Bus Rev* 66(5):121-130, 1988.

McAlvanah MF: Evaluations: an important managerial skill, *Pediatr Nurs* 14(1):75-76, 1988.

McGee KG: Making performance appraisals a positive experience, *Nurs Manage* 23(8):36-37, 1992.

Ott MJ et al: Peer interviews: sharing the hiring process, *Nurs Manage* 21(11):32-33, 1990.

Schaffer RH: Demand better results—and get them, *Harvard Bus Rev* 69(2):142-149, 1991.

Scrima DA: Assessing staff competency, *JONA* 17(2):41- 45, 1987.

Simpson DB: The performance appraisal interview: putting it all together, *Health Care Superv* 3(2):63-76, 1985.

Yochem B: Counseling: a "how-to" for new nurse managers, *Pediatr Nurs* 17(2):201-202, 1991.

Chapter 4/Communications

Baldrige L: *Leticia Baldrige's complete guide to executive manners*, New York, 1985, Rawson.

Boatwright D, Crumette BD: How to plan and conduct a patient care conference, *Nurs 87* 17(12):64, 1987.

Bradford R: Obstacles to collaborative practice, *Nurs Manage* 20(4):72I-72P, 1989.

Bushy A, Furlow L: Conflict in the operating room, *Nurs Manage, OR/Surg Procedure ed* 20(4):72a-b, 72d-e, 72h, 1989.

Burley-Allen M: *Managing assertively: how to improve your people skills*, New York, 1983, John Wiley & Sons.

Collyer ME: Resolving conflicts: leadership style sets the strategy, *Nurs Manage* 20(9):77-80, 1989.

Davidhizar R: The best approach is doing nothing, *Nurs Manage* 21(3):42-44, 1990.

Donahue M, Hebda K: How to handle troublesome employees, *RN* 47(5): 31j, 32b-h, 31-32, 1984.

Juhl N: Watch your memo manners! *Nurs Manage* 21(10):88n-p, 1990.

Keenan M, Brannon J, Dennis R: Make your meetings more productive, *Nurs Manage* 21(2):58-62, 1990.

Keenan MJ et al: Situational leadership for collaboration in health care settings, *Health Care Superv* 8(3):19-25, 1990.

Kempnich JM: Making meetings more productive, *Nurs Manage* 20(6):73-74, 1989.

Lancaster J: Creating a climate for excellence, *JONA* 15(1):16-19, 1985.

Mahan F: Patient care conferences: a model, *Nurs Manage* 19(7):60-62, 1988.

Nichols FH, Edwards MR: Are your group process skills up to par? *Nurs Health Care* 9(4):205-208, 1988.

Righ JB, Woodward-Smith MA: *Nurse manager: a practical guide to better employee relations*, Philadelphia, 1989, WB Saunders.

Russell LN: Managing the "superachiever" nurse, *Nurs Manage* 20(2): 38-39, 1989.

Schloff L, Yudkin M: *Smart speaking*, New York, 1991, Holt, Rinehart & Winston.

Schmieding NJ: Do head nurses include staff nurses in problem-solving? *Nurs Manage* 21(3):58-60, 1990.

Swansberg RC: *Management and leadership for nurse managers*, Boston, 1990, Jones & Bartlett.

Taylor MW: Listening: a key management tool, *Pediatr Nurs* 12(4):390, 422, 1991.

Turner SO: Dealing with medical staff: it's time to do it differently! *Nurs Manage* 21(2):52-53, 1990.

Chapter 5/Day-to-Day Operations

Bennett MK, Hylton JP: Modular nursing: partners in professional practice, *Nurs Manage* 21(3):20-24, 1990.

DeGroot HA: Patient classification system evaluation. I. Essential system elements, *JONA* 19(6):30-35, 1989.

DeGroot HA: Patient classification system evaluation. II. System selection and implementation, *JONA* 19(7):24-30, 1989.

Del Togno-Armanasco V, Olivas GS, Harter S: Developing an integrated nursing case management model, *Nurs Manage* 20(10):26-29, 1989.

Fletcher W: *Meetings, meetings: how to manipulate them and make them fun*, New York, 1984, William Morrow.

Giovannetti P, Thiessen M: *Patient classification for nurse staffing: criteria for selection and implementation*, Edmonton, Alberta, Canada, 1983, Alberta Association of Registered Nurses.

Glandon GL, Colbert KW, Thomasma M: Nursing delivery models and RN mix: cost implications, *Nurs Manage* 20(5):30-33, 1989.

Hass SA: Patient classification systems: a self-fulfilling prophecy, *Nurs Manage* 19(5):56-62, 1988.

Houston R: Twelve-hour shifts: answer to job satisfaction, *Nurs Manage* 21(10):88F-88H, 1990.

Huey F, Hartley S: What keeps nurses in nursing: 3,500 nurses tell their stories, *Am J Nurs* 88(2):181-188, 1988.

Jacobson E: Three new ways to deliver care, *Am J Nurs* 90(7):24-26, 1990.

Kaplow R, Outlaw E: Co-primary nursing in the intensive care unit, *Nurs Manage* 20(12):41-46, 1989.

Magaral P: Modular nursing: nurses rediscover nursing, *Nurs Manage* 18(11):98-104, 1987.

Malloch KM, Milton DA, Jobes MO: A model for differentiated nursing practice, *JONA* 20(20):20-25, 1990.

Manthey M: Primary practice partners: a nurse extender system, *Nurs Manage* 19(3):58-59, 1988.

Manthey M: Structuring work around patients, *Nurs Manage* 20(5):28-29, 1989.

Manthey M: Delivery systems and practice models: a dynamic balance, *Nurs Manage* 22(1):28-30, 1991.

Marchionno PM: Modified cyclical scheduling: a practical approach, *Nurs Manage* 18(10):60-66, 1987.

Marriner-Tomey A: *Guide to nursing management*, ed 4, St Louis, 1992, Mosby–Year Book.

Mayer GG, Madden MJ, Lawrenz E, editors: *Patient care delivery models*, Rockville, Md, 1990, Aspen.

Michael A: Team nursing and primary nursing can coexist, *Nurs Manage* 19(4):99-100, 1988.

Munson FC et al: *Nursing assignment patterns user's manual*, Ann Arbor, Mich, 1980, AUPHA Press.

Nagaprasanna BR: Patient classification systems: strategies for the 1990s, *Nurs Manage* 19(3):105-112, 1988.

Perry L: Group-practice model brings nursing unit's turnover to nil, *Mod Healthcare* 20(36):90, 1990.

Peters TJ: *Thriving on chaos*, New York, 1987, Alfred A Knopf.

Porter-O'Grady T: Shared governance for nursing, *AORN J* 53(2):458-466, 1991.

Porter-O'Grady T, Finnigan S: *Shared governance for nursing—a creative approach to professional accountability*, Rockville, Md, 1984, Aspen.

Price CA, Southerland A: Rethinking staffing patterns in critical care nursing, *Nurs Manage* 20(3):80Q-80V, 1989.

Ringl KK, Dotson L: Self-scheduling for professional nurses, *Nurs Manage* 20(2):42-44, 1989.

Satwicz MJ, Zangara A, Treston-Aurand J: Nursing and product selection = quality care, *Nurs Manage* 22(11):30-31, 1991.

Sherman RO: Team nursing revisited, *JONA* 20(11):43- 46, 1990.

Stevens BJ: *The nurse as executive,* ed 3, Rockville, Md, 1985, Aspen.

Van Slyck A: A systems approach to the management of nursing services. II. Patient classification system, *Nurs Manage* 22(4):23-25, 1991.

Wake MM: Nursing care delivery systems: status and vision, *JONA* 20(5):47-51, 1990.

Williams MA: When you don't develop your own: validation methods for patient classification systems, *Nurs Manage* 19(3):90-96, 1988.

Zander K: Nursing case management: strategic management of cost and quality outcomes, *JONA* 18(5):23-30, 1988.

Chapter 6/Effective Time Management and Productivity

Burka J, Yuen L: *Procrastination,* Reading, Mass, 1983, Addison-Wesley.

Dow C: Taming the time-eating tiger, *RN* 47(11):19-22, 1984.

Dalston JW: Effective time management techniques and guidelines. In Simendinger EA, Moore TF, Kramer M, editors: *The successful nurse executive: a guide for every nurse manager.* Ann Arbor, Mich, 1990, American College of Healthcare Executives.

Gropper EI: MBFT—management by follow-through, *Nurs Manage* 23(7): 65-66, 1992.

Harbin R: Practicing effective delegation, *Pediatr Nurs* 16(1):91-92, 1990.

Keyes R: *Timelock,* New York, 1991, Harper Collins.

Making time work for you, *Nurs 90* 20(10):144-145, 1990.

McConnell E: Ten tactics to help beat the clock, *RN* pp 47-50, Sept 1983.

Morano V: Time management: from victim to victor, *Health Care Superv* 3(1):1-12, 1984.

Oncken W, Wass D: Management time: who's got the monkey? *JONA* 20 (12):6-9, 1990.

Short B, Sumner S: Making the most of your time—by involving others, *Nurs 90* pp 99-104, Jan 1990.

Smith H, Besnette F: Effective time management: the forgotten administrative and nursing supervisor art, *Hosp Top* 56(1):32-37, 1978.

Chapter 7/Budgeting Basics

Felteau A: Budget variance analysis and justification, *Nurs Manage* 23(2): 40-41, 1992.

Kerfoot K, Rohe D: Nursing management considerations: innovations for nurse managers to improve productivity, *Nurs Econ* 7(4):228-230, 1989.

Loevinsohn HT: A new perspective on scheduling: freedom and cost control, *Nurs Manage* 23(7):56-61, 1992.

Porter-O'Grady T: *Nursing finance— budgeting strategies for a new age,* Rockville, Md, 1987, Aspen.

Schwartz WB, Mendelson DN: Hospital cost containment in the 1980s: hard lessons learned and prospects for the 1990s, *N Engl J Med* 324 (15):1037-1042, 1991.

Tzirides E, Waterstraat V, Chamberlin W: Managing the budget with a fluctuating census, *Nurs Manage* 22 (3):80B-80H, 1991.

Wilburn D: Budget response to volume variability, *Nurs Manage* 23(2):42-44, 1992.

Chapter 8/Legal Issues and Risk Management

Bergerson SR: More about charting with a jury in mind, *Nurs 88* 18(4):50-88, 1988.

Bradford EB: Preventing malpractice suits, *Nurs 88* 18(9):63-64, 1988.

Creighton H: More about floating, *Nurs Manage* 18(8):17-18, 1987.

Cushing M: The legal side: accepting or rejecting an assignment. I. Are you abandoning your patients? *Am J Nurs* 88(11):1470-1476, 1988.

Feutz SA: How to cope with understaffing, *Nurs 91* 21(8):54-55, 1991.

Fiesta J: Agency nurses—whose liability? *Nurs Manage* 21(3):16-17, 1990.

Fiesta J: The nursing shortage: whose liability problem? Part II, *Nurs Manage* 21(2):22-23, 1990.

Guarriello DL: When doctor's orders aren't the best medicine, *RN* 47(5):19-20, 1984.

Luquire R: Nursing risk management, *Nurs Manage* 20(10):56-58, 1989.

Mandell M: Practical ways to survive a lawsuit, *Nurs 92* 22(8):56-57, 1992.

Northrup CE: Refusing unsafe work assignments, *Nurs Outlook* 35(6):32, 1987.

Chapter 9/Quality Assessment and Improvement

Arikian VL: Total quality management: applications to nursing service, *JONA* 21(6):46-50, 1991.

Beyers M: Quality: the banner of the 1980's, *Nurs Clin North Am* 23(3):617-623, 1988.

Bushy A: Quality assurance in rural hospitals, *JONA* 21(10):34-39, 1991.

Del Bueno D, Vincent PM: Organizational culture: how important is it? *JONA* 16(10):15-20, 1986.

Gillem TR: Deming's 14 points and hospital quality: responding to the consumer's demand for the best value health care, *J Nurs Qual Assur* 2(3):70-78, 1988.

Harrington HJ: *The improvement process: how America's leading companies improve quality*, New York, 1987, McGraw-Hill.

Harris SH et al: A problem-focused quality assurance program, *Nurs Manage* 20(2):54-60, 1989.

Hoesing H, Kirk R: Common sense quality management, *JONA* 20(10):10-15, 1990.

Jacobson E: Three new ways to deliver care, *Am J Nurs* 90(7):24-26, 1990.

Joint Commission on the Accreditation of Healthcare Organizations (JCAHO): *Accreditation manual for home care* Chicago, Ill, 1991, JCAHO.

Joint Commission on the Accreditation of Healthcare Organizations (JCAHO): *Accreditation manual for hospitals*, vol 1, Standards, Chicago, Ill, 1992, JCAHO.

Kramer M: Trends to watch at the magnet hospital, *Nurs 90* 20(6):67-74, 1990.

Micheletti JA, Shlala TJ: Evolving quality assurance initiatives in home healthcare, *Nurs Manage* 20(8):24-28, 1989.

Mitchell K: Hospital knows best? *Nurs Econ* 5(6):266, 291, 1987.

New NA: Quality measurement: quick, easy and unit-based, *Nurs Manage* 20(10):50-51, 1989.

New N, New JR: Quality assurance that works, *Nurs Manage* 20(6):21-24, 1989.

Poe SS, Will JC: Quality nurse-patient outcomes: a framework for nursing practice, *J Nurs Qual Assur* 2(1):29-38, 1987.

Porter AL: Assuring quality through staff nurse performance, *Nurs Clin North Am* 23(3):649-655, 1988.

Robbins CL, Robbins WA: What nurse managers should know about sampling techniques, *Nurs Manage* 20 (6):46-48, 1989.

Schoeder P: Directions and dilemmas in nursing quality assurance, *Nurs Clin North Am* 23(3):657-664, 1988.

Schoeder P, Maibusch R: *Nursing quality assurance: a unit based approach*, Rockville, Md, 1984, Aspen.

Summers P et al: Quality management: program design, an interdisciplinary approach, *Nurs Clin North Am* 23 (3):665-670, 1988.

Chapter 10/Taking Care of Yourself and Staff

Albrecht TL, Halsey J: Supporting the staff nurse under stress, *Nurs Manage* 22(7):60-61, 64, 1991.

Bennett S, Robertson R, Moss P: Education: learning the pitfalls of code-pendency, *Nurs Manage* 23(2):80B-80H, 1992.

Casey JL: Counseling nurse managers, *Nurs Manage* 20(9):52-53, 1989.

Cauthorne-Lindstrom C, Hrabe D: Co-dependent behaviors in managers: a script for failure, *Nurs Manage* 21 (2):34-39, 1990.

Fortman R: Staff support groups: what works, what doesn't, *Hospice* 1(1):23-25, 1990.

Guntzelman J: Making frustration work for you, *Nurs 90,* 20(12):85-89, 1990.

Kaplan SM: The nurse as change agent, *Pediatr Nurs* 16(6):603-605, 1990.

Lee BS: Humor relations for nurse managers, *Nurs Manage* 21(5):86, 88, 90, 1990.

Nicholson LG: Stress management in nursing, *Nurs Manage* 21(4):53-55, 1990.

Patton J: Addicted nurses, *J Pract Nurs* 37(4):38-40, 1987.

Selbach KH: Chemical dependency in nursing, *AORN J* 52(3), 1990.

Chapter 11/When Bad Things Happen to Good Managers

Betancourt EK: Job sharing in nursing management: it can work, *Nurs Manage* 21(1):47-49, 1990.

Bramson RM: *Coping with difficult people,* New York, 1981, Ballantine Books.

Collyer ME: Resolving conflicts: leadership style sets the strategy, *Nurs Manage* 20(9):77-80, 1989.

King P: *Never work for a jerk,* New York, 1987, Dell.

O'Neil KK: The head nurse's managerial role, *Nurs Manage* 20(6):39-41, 1989.

Perlman D, Takacs G: The 10 stages of change, *Nurs Manage* 21(4):33-38, 1990.

Chapter 12/The Nurse Manager in Homecare and Hospice

A statement on the scope of home health nursing practice, Kansas City, 1992, The American Nurses Association.

Health Insurance Manual-11, Home Health Agency Manual Washington DC, 1990, Government Printing Office.

Joint Commission on Accreditation of Healthcare Organizations: *1993 joint commission accreditation manual for home care,* Oakbrook Terrace, Ill, 1992, The JCAHO.

Marrelli, T.M. *Handbook of home health standards and documentation guidelines for reimbursement,* St. Louis, 1991, Mosby.

Marrelli TM. *Nursing documentation handbook*, St. Louis, 1992, Mosby.

Sherry D: The incredible, F-L-E-X-I-B-L-E nurse, *Nurs 85*, 15(12):72, 1985.

Standards of home health nursing practice, Kansas City, 1986, The American Nurses Association.

Stanhope M, Knollmueller R: *Handbook of community and home health nursing*, St. Louis, 1992, Mosby.

Woerner L, Feldstein KC: *Scheduling home health care personnel*, New York, 1988, John Wiley & Sons.

Chapter 13/Where To From Here?

Bolles RN: *What color is your parachute?* Berkeley, Calif, 1992, Ten Speed Press.

Butler J, Parsons RJ: Hospital perceptions of job satisfaction, *Nurs Manage* 20(8):45-48, 1989.

Carroll MF: *Credentialing in nursing: contemporary developments and trends*, Kansas City, Mo, 1987, American Nurse's Association.

Cosgray RE et al: Getting started on your first manuscript, *Hosp Top*, 67(5): 28-32, 1989.

Fisher P, Vry W: *Getting to yes: negotiating agreement without giving in*, New York, 1981, Penguin Books.

Flores DW: Marketing yourself in an interview, *Nurs 92* 22(8):100-102, 1992.

Kaplan SM: The nurse as change agent, *Pediatr Nurs* 16(6):603-695, 1990.

Krouse HJ, Holleran SD: Nurse managers and clinical nursing research, *Nurs Manage* 23(7):62-64, 1992.

Newcomb BJ, Murphy PA: The curriculum vitae—what it is and what it is not, *Nurs Outlook* 27(9):580-583, 1979.

O'Connor P: Resumes: opening the door, *Nurs Econ* 2:428-431, 1984.

Pearlman D, Takacs GJ: The 10 stages of change, *Nurs Manage* 21(4):33-38, 1990.

Perry L: Nursing supervisors continue to lead climb up the ladder, *Mod Healthcare* 21(21):27-34, 1991.

Sher B: *Wishcraft*, New York, 1983, Random House.

Taylor T: Healthcare marketing and the nurse manager, *Nurs Manage* 21(5):84-85, 1990.

Index

Budget variance report, 154
Budgeting, 134-163
  assets and, 137
  break-even analysis and, 158-159
  capital expansion and, 137-138
  case management and, 144-145
  cost-based reimbursement and, 135-136
  costs and, 149-151
  diagnostic-related groups and, 135
  discounted services and, 143
  financial performance reports and, 139,
    140
  financial standards and, 158
  fiscal management and, 136-137
  indicators for, 153-155
  insurance and, 140-143
  liabilities and, 137
  net worth and, 137
  nurse manager in, 151-153
  payor mix and, 143-144
  process of, 145-149
  productivity measurement and, 156-158
  productivity ratings and, 160
  profit and, 137
  public perception of hospitals and,
    138-139
  reinvestment and, 137-138
  styles of, 145-149
  terminology in, 162-163
  total quality management and, 134-135
  trends in, 160
Burden of proof, 185

C

Camaraderie, 273-274
Capacity, informed consent and, 174-175
Capital budget, 146-147
Capital expansion, 137-138
Capitation, 142
Captain of ship doctrine, 185
Care
  for dying patient, 213
  patient-centered, 96
  standards of
    negligence and, 166
    quality assessment and, 203
Care team model, professionally
    advanced, 95-96
Career opportunities, 289-308
  choices in, 292-293
  identifying skills and, 293-295
  interviewing and, 297-304
  job acceptance and, 306-307
  job satisfaction assessment and, 289-292

Career opportunities—cont'd
  marketing yourself and, 293
  negotiating and, 304-306
  networking and, 296
  resignation and, 307-308
  resumes and, 296-297
Case management, 94-95, 144-145
Cause
  of action, 185
  negligence and, 168
  proximate, 191
Centralized scheduling, 103
Certificate of Need, 265
Certification, 108-109, 293-294
  in homecare, 271
Certiorari, writ of, 193
Challenge, 121
Change
  attitudes and, 121-122
  identification of need for, 261-262
  stress and, 2
Chaplaincy service checklist, 17
Chart
  audit of, 197
  quality assessment and, 201
Checklist
  for chaplaincy services, 17
  for data processing, 17
  for dietary or food service, 17
  for documentation, 279-280
  for education, 20-21
  financial, 17-18
  for home health care, 19-20
  for human resource management, 18
  for laboratory services, 18
  for medical record, 18
  for orientation, 13, 53-55
  for radiologic service, 19
  for rehabilitation service, 19
  for services, 17-21
  for staff education, 20-21
Chemically dependent employee, 237-238
Choices, career, 292-293
Climate, communication, 74
Clinical conference, 113-114
Clinical expertise, 42
Clinical record assessment, 201-202
Clinical rounds, 114-115
Coaching, 56-60
Coercive power, 6
Collaboration, 68
Commitment, 122
Committee, quality, 200
Common law, 185

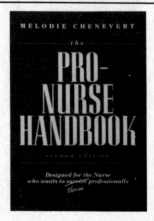
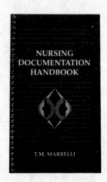